CHAKRA

ENTREPRENEUR

MANAGE YOUR CHAKRA
TO GROW YOUR BUSINESS

CHAKRA ENTREPRENEUR

MANAGE YOUR CHAKRA
TO GROW YOUR BUSINESS

Authored by
Manika Singh

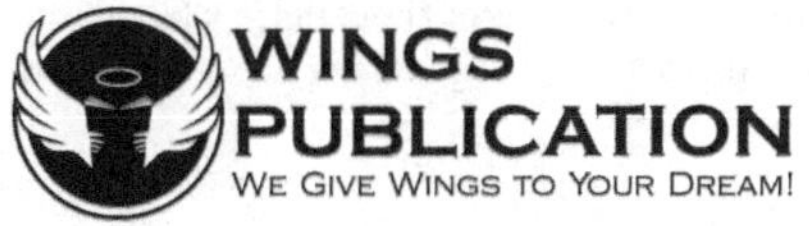

Disclaimer

This book has been published with all reasonable efforts taken to make the material error-free after the consent of the author. This book is sold subject to the condition that it shall not, by way of trade or otherwise, be lent, resold, or otherwise circulated without the copyright owner's prior written consent in any form of binding or cover other than that in which it is published and without a similar condition including this condition being imposed on the subsequent purchaser and without limiting the rights under copyright reserved above, no part of this publication maybe reproduced, stored in or introduced into a retrieval system or transmitted in any form or by any other means without the permission of the copyright owner.

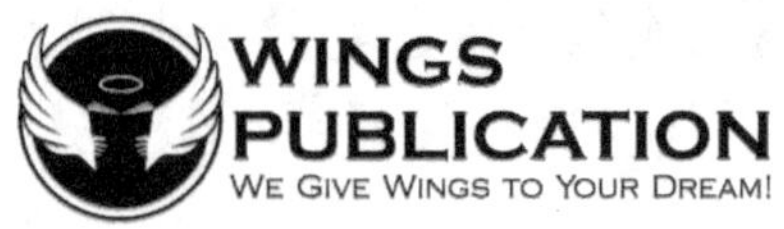

Registered Office- 907-Sneh Nagar, Sapna Sangeeta Road,
Agrasen Square, Indore – 452001 (M.P.), India
Website: http://www.wingspublication.com
Email: mybook@wingspublication.com

First Published by WINGS PUBLICATION 2022
Copyright © Manika Singh 2022

Title: **CHAKRA ENTREPRENEUR**
All Rights Reserved.

Content

Acknowledgement

The completion of this book could not have been possible without the participation and assistance of so many people whose names may not all be enumerated. Their contributions are sincerely appreciated and gratefully acknowledged. However, I would like to express my deep appreciation and indebtedness to

My Guru Anodea Judith, for showing me the path of success. Her book "Wheels of Life" and her teachings opened my perspective about many things related to Chakra and its application.

To Louise Hay who taught me that you can heal your life and achieve health, wealth and success with right attitude.

My husband Kailash for his endless support and understanding spirit during case presentation.

To all relatives, friends and others who in one way or another shared their support. Thank You!!

Above all to the Great Almighty, the author of knowledge and wisdom for his countless love.

Preface

Few months back while visiting my doctor's clinic, I noticed the doctor's logo being displayed there. Have you ever seen the doctor's logo? Here it is for your reference.

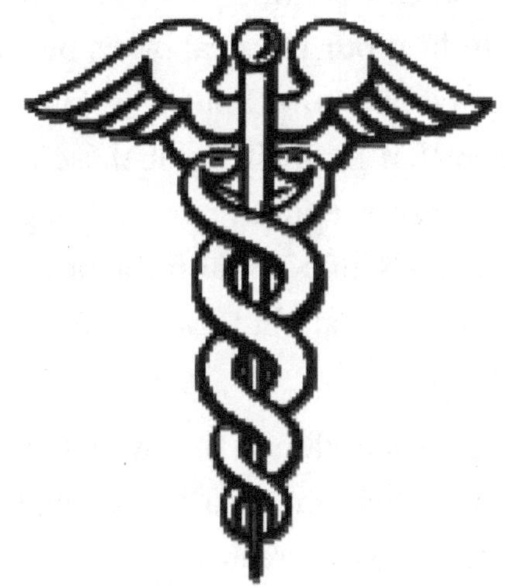

In a flash, I thought that this doctor is a kundalini vidya fan and have put this logo as a symbol of admiration. But then I realized that this is actually a doctor's logo. But there is resemblance of the logo to our ancient wisdom of Kundalini symbol. Take a look, isn't it almost the same.

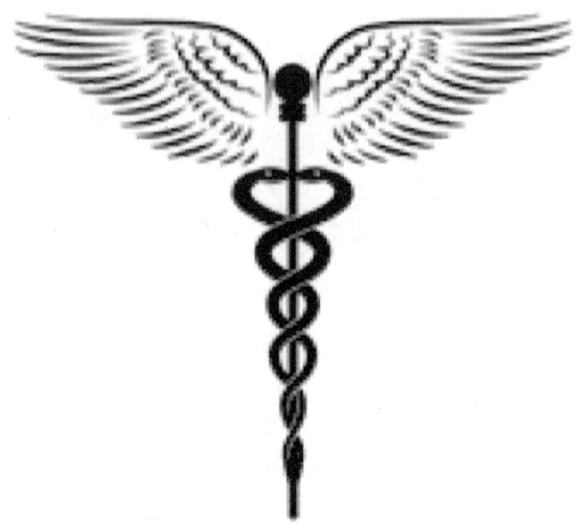

Medical advancement definitely focuses around the physical realms and how to heal our physical body, but the total healing process cannot be complete without emotional attributes. Is it a coincidence then that the pairing of these two snakes of the caduceus (that you can see on the doctor's logo) are extremely similar to the channels of Kundalini, a power that has great potential to not only heal, but raise the awareness of our consciousness?

We humans are the storehouse of power. Our entire body has an electric field. Anywhere there's a nerve cell, there's electricity. It's more concentrated and greatest around our head because that's where the bulk of our nerve cells are. Any time you've felt the shock of static electricity, or used a touch-sensitive screen, you've proven that you have an electric field.

So, nothing mysterious about that part.

Being an electric field, all those overlying electric wave patterns that comprise your brain waves are governed by the same equations governing the electromagnetic spectrum, light, particles and everything else in the universe. The light seen coming from a star and the energy of your mind are one and the same type.

Your thoughts are formed in this electric field. The measurable perturbations and disturbances in the brain's overall electric field are your actual thoughts racing through your mind. As you read this Book, the thoughts you are thinking of, the words your mind is processing, are all electrical impulses that can be measured if you had a few wires hooked up between your head and a machine. So, thoughts are energy, the same as everything else.

This subject always intrigued me and forced me to dig deeper more and more into this vast learning.

Can this power be utilized properly to heal ourselves not only physically but emotionally, mentally, spiritually, financially? Can we improve our relationships, health, wealth and create a dream life that we always wish and desire for?

The answer that I got, after tremendous research was a YES… but how? I mean, I want to think positive and good thoughts. We all want to have positive thoughts, but why a negative seed crops up and make it a big tree of anxiety, worry, tension, fear?

As an Entrepreneur I have failed in 3 businesses and made huge losses. I started my business journey with enthusiastic mindset, did all the proper planning on the excel sheet with the numbers and figures which were pointing towards profits, but down the lane things started to take a toll. Sales were not happening, money was not coming, clients were unhappy and my balance sheet was a horror story altogether.

Now, when I look back, I could notice the same pattern of mistakes being repeated by me in all the 3 businesses of course with version 1.0, 2.0 and 3.0. I took a break and went on a sabbatical, where I connected the dots. This made me released that to come out of the repeated pattern mistakes, I had to reprogram my inbuilt software programming. I wanted to understand the power beyond the hard work and smart work.

Have you also ever felt that even the most calculated strategy of yours can still fetch you a mediocre result?

A great idea, hard work, good counsel, research, and inspiration from others are great ways to find success in business. But sometimes, try as we might, we just seem… blocked…

The reasons the results didn't happen may be because you actually weren't ready...

Maybe your personal energy, weren't sufficient enough to take you through the roadblocks. Maybe you are charged at the outer level, but inside you have anxiety about sales, money, your product/services, your confidence, competitors, your mission and vision.

Our business is an energetic reflection of ourselves.

Energy flows through a business, much as it flows through a body. And things like momentum need that energy to ignite into tornadoes of business.

Strategies will come and go, however: Your ability to stay connected within & feel empowered is the #1 strategy that WILL remain the same.

So, while everyone is telling you what to do and how to do it, make sure you take time out regularly to do the inner work that's required to stay connected.

You may be noticing that business has never actually been about just 'selling a product'. Rather, it's been about connecting to the emotions of your audience and sharing with them how you understand them first and foremost, and then how you can help them.

The deeper you can connect to your personal energies, the deeper and more powerful you will be able to connect with your tribe on an emotional level, and you'll be able to really ignite your business.

This book is an attempt to tap into the energy of self, make you understand the patterns that is creating the blockages in your business and how you can rectify it from within.

This book is written in a simple language for even my 10-year kid to understand the concept. I myself don't like jargons and difficult things, and have avoided it all together.

Many entrepreneurs initially are completely shocked to listen to Business advise and spiritual advise been given together. But the truth is if you align yourself, lot of your miseries in life will be solved. And Business being the bigger representation of you, will be on the track of growth and success. This I am talking from my personal experience.

Start to explore, there is always more to learn and a new unfolding to occur for you - no matter where you are on the business success ladder.

Enjoy the journey!

Chapter 1

YOUR BUSINESS IS AN ENERGETIC REFLECTION OF YOU

Have you ever looked at your business from this perspective, that it's a reflection of you? It's an extension of you. It's communicating with you. It's growing you and growing with you.

Your energy, willpower, motivation, attitude decides the future of your Business. Everything falls into place and beings to flow, when you are in **balanced energy.** We human beings are a mass of energy and everything around us is energy. This book you are reading, the chair you are sitting, your house, your laptop, your money. Yes, everything is energy.

Our famous Albert Einstein stated **E=MC2.** Which means that Mass (matter) can be converted into energy. We are mass and energy. Everything around us is made up of vibrating particles and energy. Even the smallest cell in our body is vibrating into energy. These vibrations are invisible to us because they're too small to see with naked eyes.

We humans are electrical beings. Electrical signals travel throughout our brain and down to our muscles, telling them when and how to move. Signals from the brain can easily be measured with an electroencephalograph (EEG), and measured from the muscles with an electromyograph (EMG). Because electricity flows through us, we are conductors.

When electricity moves through a conductor, such as a wire, an electromagnetic field (EMF) is created around it. Because we are conductors, it follows that we have an EMF, a field of energy, around our bodies. Some people call it aura.

The health of our aura is directly connected to the health of our physical body, the mind, and our emotional wellbeing. It acts as a shield around our body. They are our transmitters and receptors, constantly receiving and releasing frequencies. The energies we are in while we take action in our business or any task, can have a direct impact on what we get as a result. That's why it's so important to balance ourselves as they relate to business self-sabotages and blocks.

There are many energy centres in our auric body which is in the form of wheel, circle or chakra. If our energy centres are balanced, the information flows freely and we are prepared to act in a way that serves our best interest and keeps us healthy. If the flow of energy gets blocked, it stagnates and starts to create toxicity in our bodies in the form of negative thoughts, feelings and physical manifestations. Imagine a flowing river that gets blocked and stops flowing. When that happens, it turns into a swamp—moldy, nasty, diseased and stinky. Well, the same thing happens in our body. And when one energy gets blocked, (it's common for it to get blocked) the chain reaction wreaks havoc on our mindset (negative thinking, self-doubt, worry), our emotions (depression, frustration, jealousy, anger, fear) and our bodies (aches, pains and disease).

On the other hand, when our energies are open and flowing,

we have the mental capacity to perform business tasks at an optimum level. We are enthusiastic and confident; we give and receive love openly and we are optimistic about the future. We feel emotionally capable and ready to take on all of the action steps required to reach our business goals, including stepping outside our comfort zone, feeling confident in our abilities and taking on new projects with faith and courage. And when we are physically able to rise to the challenges of business without stress and anxiety, we are able to wake up each day with energy, passion and vitality. Reaching our goals becomes fun and easy.

A few signs that your energy centres (chakras) are blocked or imbalanced:

- **Stressed** – you have a hard time relaxing or being in the present moment.

- **Worried all the time** – you can't seem to shut your mind off and may even be losing sleep.

- **Anxiety** – your heart beats fast all day long, you're always racing the clock and you're nervous about what the future holds.

- **Unmotivated** – you're just going through the motions, without any real passion or drive.

- **Depressed** – you are losing hope and starting to feel like your situation may never change.

- **Overwhelmed** – no matter how much you try to manage your time; you can't seem to get ahead.

- **Frustrated** – you aren't making the progress that you want to make in your business.

- **Doubtful** – you are questioning your abilities to reach the goals you set for yourself.

When these feelings are present, your mindset will start to become affected too. You may start to think, *"Am I really good at this? Am I capable? I probably shouldn't do this. I should probably back off. It's never going to work anyway."* And the more we think those limiting thoughts, the more stressed, anxious, depressed, and sad we become, and then we think even more negative thoughts and the cycle continues until we start to physically show signs of disease. So, it's vital to make sure that we are paying attention to the red flags that notify us when a chakra may be imbalanced before the chaos is out of control.

I am going to break down each chakra, individually, so that you can recognize which one to get back to a state of balance and flow.

Your blocked Chakras can be the reason behind you:

- Not making income in your business

- Not attracting your dream clients

- Having a lack of inspiration, motivation or desire to work on building your business

- Communicating your message, your programs and your pricing with ease

- Fear and lack of energy to take action and accomplish your goals

• Unclear vision and clarity about future

and that's just to name a few!

To tell you problems don't sprout up in a day or two. Because of our conditioning, old pattern or beliefs we have built our energy systems in this way, which creates hurdles in us achieving the desired results.

Let's understand what is the relations between our chakras, our emotions, our belief system and our body, which ultimately affects our BUSINESS.

Why we do certain things or why we are not able to do somethings!!!

Chapter 2

RELATIONSHIP BETWEEN BODY AND MIND

Have you heard this phrase **"We are what we think about all day long"?** Every thought we think is creating our future. The point of power is always in the present moment.

But are we using our power to the fullest?? No… Because most of us suffer from the disease of self-hatred, criticism and guilt. We keep blaming ourselves. The bottom line for many of us is **"I am not good".**

By continuously repeating these negative thoughts …….We are first creating illness in our mind and then transporting that illness in our body.

The feeling of resentment, criticism, anger and guilt are the most damaging patterns. These feelings eat us from Inside.

Next time just notice how your body feels when you are angry. The emotion of Anger erupts from our mind and then engulfs our physical body. Your heart rate, blood pressure and respiration increase, the body temperature rises and your skin starts to perspires. Anger is an emotional energy state inside us which affects our body outside.

Not only anger, just notice the effect of other emotional energies erupting inside us and affecting our body. If we are happy our body vibrates with positivity, it brings smile on our face and we feel calm, peaceful and relaxed.

It is said that releasing resentment can even dissolve **cancer?**

For our good health we must release our negative emotions as it affects both our body and mind.

This is I call **"Emotional Health Quotient".**

Why it is vital to understand the Emotional Health Quotient?

You need to know and understand your emotional quotient to work with yourself at the root base level. For example: Is attracting money a problem, why you are not good at sales, do you fear failure or criticism. Why do you take certain action or procrastinate some decision making?

Let's understand this -

We human beings live in 2 planes:

(1) Physical Plane which consists of our body. Which is tangible – we can see, touch, feel, smell etc. We know this plane very well as we can see it and most of us work only on this plane. Going to office daily, pushing ourselves hard to complete the task, working unlimitedly in front of our laptops etc.

(2) Energy Plane which consists of our emotions, feelings, attitude, behaviour, beliefs etc. Many people don't talk about this or doesn't do anything about this. But to tell you the fact, our emotional health plays a crucial role in attracting the results and outcomes in our lives

Our overall wellbeing includes physical, emotional, intellectual, social, and spiritual aspects. When they all are in balance and alignment, human beings thrive. Each of these areas of life influences each other's.

What is Emotional health is a person's ability to accept and manage his/her feelings. Someone who is emotionally healthy can allow their emotions to be digestible. Life will throw problems at you but it is your response to those troubles which will decide your emotional wellbeing. We all have a storehouse or warehouse of emotions, which is stored as per the childhood conditioning, repeated patterns, behaviours or belief system. Any incident occurs and your mental system will pick up the emotions as per the previous incidents. Example if you are stuck in a traffic during office hours. What response you will give? Will your emotion system pick up the anger response, because that is stored as a behaviour or belief system in your database or will give you a fear response, as you might be late for the meeting?

Imagine that when you are emotionally down or disbalanced like anger or frustration can you put in 100% effort in your work or anywhere. You will drain so much of your energies and ultimately will spoil your moment or day.

When you have positively charged energy and emotions you carry yourself with a sense of confidence, self-acceptance, and openness. You will automatically start making healthier decisions and choices for yourself.

How do we create our Beliefs and Emotional Health?

Now an important question comes that how do we learn

these emotions. How did we learn to think about ourselves and about our world? This goes back to our childhood age. We treat ourselves the way our parents treated us. We scold and punish ourselves in the same way. You can almost hear the words when you listen. We also love and encourage ourselves the same way.

"You never do anything right." "It's all your fault." How often have you said this to yourself? We learn our belief systems as very little child and then we move through life creating experiences to match our beliefs. Look back in your own life and notice how often you have gone through the same experience.

Just as computer programming has source code, our emotions and belief also have one. As a source code these emotions and belief systems are developed in our system when we were growing up and have deep rooted its base in our programming. Whatever we do, have and say is all governed by this backend programme.

But there is a way to change these beliefs and programming. Of course, it will not happen in a day or two. You will have to deliberately put in efforts for the change of the programming, but yes there is a way out.

Are you feeling lonely, are you sad, are you afraid, do you think that you are not good enough? Become aware of your emotions, understand the triggers and then divert that energy into positive. Which we will learn in the further chapters how to balance your emotions.

We need to understand when this belief system was developed and how does it affect us. We will have to heal ourselves. Healing works by bringing body, mind and energy together.

Chapter 3

CHAKRAS UNDERSTANDING

How did we go from being a tiny perfect baby to being a person who has problems and feels unworthy and unlovable to one degree or another?

The answer is in our ancient India culture – our Chakras.

What are Chakras – Energy Centres?

Chakras means wheel. They are the energy centres in your body. These spinning energy wheels correspond to certain nerve bundles and major organs of our body. You can think of it as chambers in our body. Just like the chambers of your home, like kitchen, bedroom, living room, bathroom etc. Each chamber is designed to receive different kind of energy. When you come home from a grocery store you put your food in the kitchen. You don't take it to the bathroom. That kitchen is designed to handle the food, designed to let you prepare it, assimilate it, eat it and place to put the garbage so you can throw unwanted stuff out.

Similarly, each of the chambers in our body is designed to receive and handle a particular kind of energy and how **we receive it, assimilate it, store it** or express it has to do with the health and energy of that chakra. So, when we are healing different chakras, we are balancing it. The chakra system originated in

India between 1500 and 500 BC in the oldest text called the Vedas.

The content of the chakras is formed largely by repeated patterns from our actions in day-to-day life. Repeated movements and habits create world around us.

These chakras exist within the subtle body or auric/energy body, interpenetrating the physical body. The subtle body is the nonphysical psychic body that is superimposed on our physical bodies. It can be measured as electromagnetic force fields within and around all living creatures. We consider who we are to be in the form of just "THE BODY", which is actually an intricate system of physiological process.

If you would like to experience what an energy body feels like, the following is a simple exercise for opening the hand chakras and experience the energy:

Extend both arms out in front of you, parallel to the floor with elbows straight.

Turn one hand up and one hand down. Now quickly open and close your hands a dozen times or so.

Reverse your palms and repeat. This opens the hand chakras.

To feel their energy, open your hands and slowly bring your palms together, starting about 2 feet apart.

When your hands are about four inches apart you should be able to feel a subtle ball of energy, like a magnetic field, floating between your palms. If you tune in closely, you may even be able to feel it spinning.

After a few moments the sensation will subside, but it can be repeated by opening and closing the palms again as above.

How do Chakras Work?

Chakras are the vortex of energy spinning at the core of the body. They are the gates that mediates between the inner and outer world. They act as a barrier to keep things from coming inside us or somethings going out.

Chakras contain programme and programme start from the birth.

Some of the programming is conscious like the language we speak, things we believe. And most of it are unconscious. Programme that governs our behaviour our thoughts. The purpose here is to make unconscious conscious so that we choose wisely.

For example, the emotional experience of fear, related to the first chakra. Fear affects our body in certain ways. We feel butterflies in our stomach, our breath is short and our voice and hands may shake. These physical characteristics betray our lack of confidence in dealing with the world and may lead others to treat us in a negative way, perpetuating our fear. This fear may have its roots in an unresolved childhood experience, yet still rules our behaviour.

To work with the chakras is to heal ourselves of old constricting patterns lodged in the body or the mind, or habitual behaviour.

While chakras are interdependent with the nervous system and endocrine systems, they are not synonymous with any portion of the physical body, but exist within the subtle body. Yet their effect upon the physical body is strong. I believe that chakras generate the shape and behaviour of the physical body, much as the mind influences our emotions. An excessive 3rd chakra would exhibit a big tight belly, a constricted 5th Chakra results in tight shoulders or sore throat, a poor connection through the first chakra may show up in skinny legs or bad knees.

These chakras are the lens of looking at the life – like looking at our survival issue, your emotional issue, your power issue, your relationship issue, your communication issue, your imagination, your wisdom. Looking at all these different aspects of your life. From instinctual behaviour to consciously planned strategies, from emotions to artistic creations, the chakras are the master programs that govern our life, loves, learning and illumination.

Chakras have locations in our body and through that we look at the elements in each chakra – **Earth, Water, Fire, Air, Sound, Light and thought**. We look at these elements and which part of the body they are located, what that part of the body is doing and creating emotions and from that it creates a full physiological system that creates your life.

Like Survival issues coming from this part of your life, emotional issues coming from this part of your life. I started to put them together and build up a whole physiological schema. And have started seeing amazing results in the correction of many life issues.

When energy gets blocked, we get emotional and physical issues in our systems. For example, we want to have a big car or house for us, that's what our vision is, but we have a scarcity issue which is a problem of root chakra then in that case the energy gets blocked up in the system and we will not be able to manifest the dream. There will be knots (knots of resistance) that the energy can't get through and the current will not be liberating. We will first have to harmonise these chakras so that the flow of energy is smooth all the way from bottom of the chakra to the top.

Chakras are energy centres a response to what happens in your life. When you feel a threat, your energy may increase in order to deal with the threat or it may scare you so much that you say I am not here. You would want to avoid it. **That's creates an excessive coping strategy of deficient coping strategy.** You may have a deficient heart chakra that just doesn't want to deal with relationship or you may have an excessive heart chakra that needs to be the centre of attention all the time. So, we look at the blocks to understand the emotional behaviour pattern and then accordingly comes the treatment.

An excessive chakra energy needs to get rid of the energy or charge and deficient chakra needs to take in. It needs to expand and really receive. When we talk about chakra balancing, we have to balance the excessive or deficient charge.

By balancing our chakras, we can balance our life.

- We can release limiting, unproductive patterns of the past and replace them with new habits and behaviours.

- To mend the wounds of childhood that are lodged in the physical, emotional and mental programming.

- And finally, to take your inner work into your outer world.

The structure of this book is to understand various chakras and how various programme are built in our system. Things we are taught, things we have gone through and experienced, how we dealt with that, what are the defences that allowed us to survive, they taught us what we believe. They have put those programmes into our nervous system, even the structure/posture of your body.

The trouble is we have bugs in our programme and sometimes

we need to upgrade those programmes in order to work in the modern system. We need to clear old limiting beliefs that comes in the way of proper functioning.

We will clear the blockages of the 7 chakras so that the energy system in the body flows smoothly and we can live a happy, healthy and prosperous life. We have all the energy to take all the wonders of the life and live life perfectly in all the arenas of life.

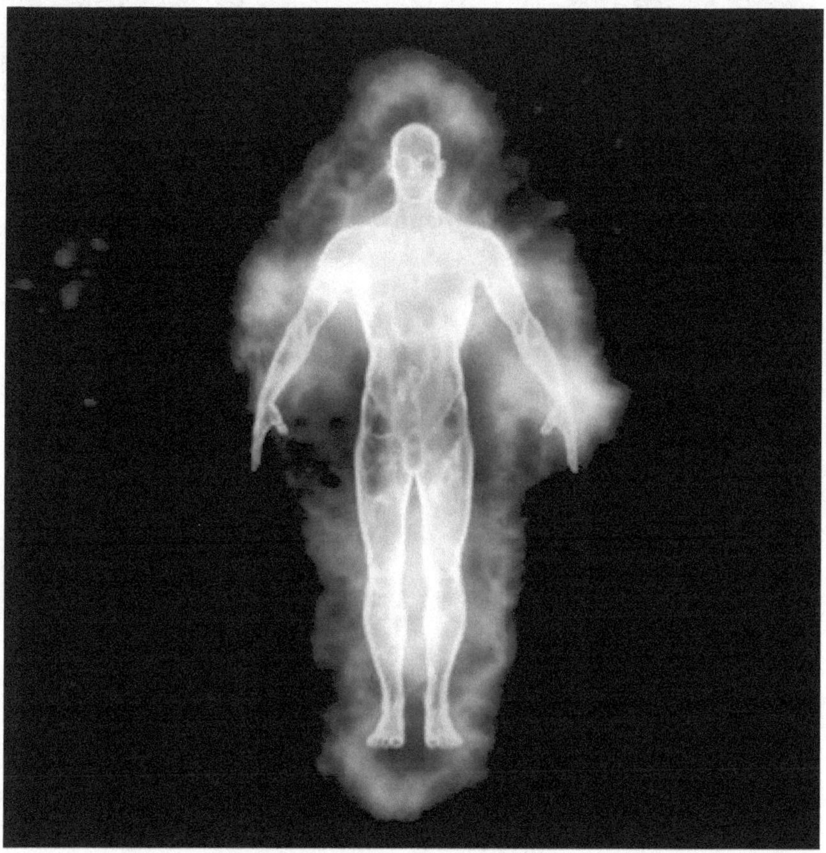

Aura of Human Body

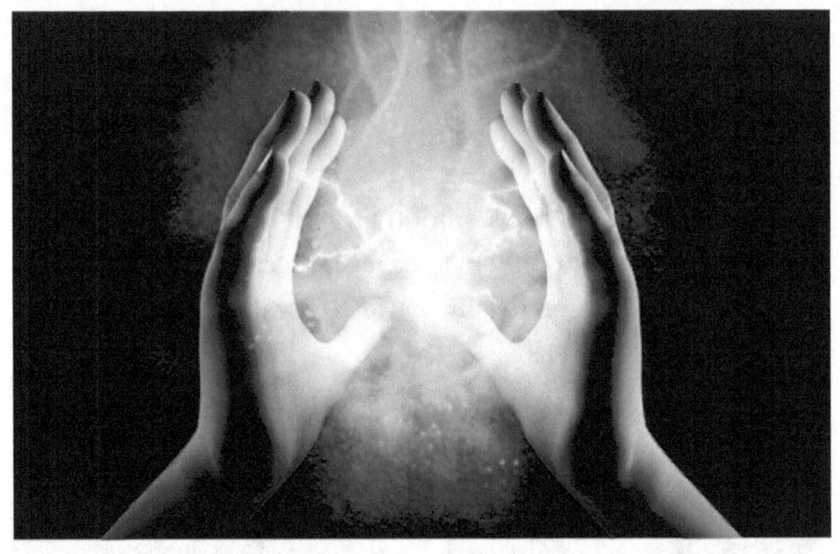

Aura around our Hand

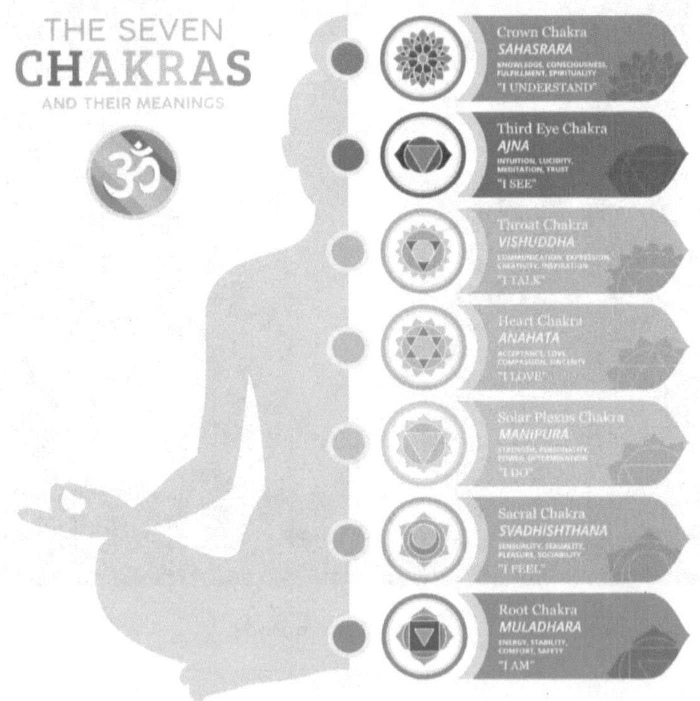

Exercise

Look at the self-assessment and become aware of which chakras need more attention

PRE-ASSESSMENT

Pre-Assessment: Overall Chakra Health

Before you start understanding the chakras and its disbalance, it's important to gauge your baseline chakra health. The pre-assessment below is helpful for two reasons:

1. It will help clarify what areas you need to focus on.

2. It will help set a reference point for yourself, so you can later evaluate which areas you've developed.

There is an assessment at the back of the book as well, rate yourself again to see how much you have grown. Then, calculate the difference of your pre and post assessments.

If there are areas where you still feel stuck, areas that didn't change that much, then you know where you need to do deeper work, or apply the practices longer or more diligently. Don't beat yourself up about it, just keep up the efforts. They will pay off in the long run.

Instructions

Use the rating scale below to rate yourself on each statement.

Not at all	A little	Sometimes	Often	Most of the Time
1	2	3	4	5

First Chakra: Root

1. _______ I have trouble finding or holding my ground.

2. _______ I'm not at ease in my body.

3. _______ I have health challenges.

4. _______ I hate to exercise.

5. _______ I struggle with food, diet, or weight.

6. _______ I never seem to have enough money to live comfortably.

7. _______ I feel disconnected with nature and the earth.

First Chakra Total = __________

Second Chakra: Sacral

1. _______ I have trouble knowing what I feel.

2. _______ Some people think I'm overly emotional.

3. _______ I find sexuality to be challenging for me.

4. _______ Life just isn't a whole lot of fun.

5. _______ My body doesn't move very freely.

6. _______ I have trouble knowing what I want and need.

7. _______ If I do know what I want, I'm scared to ask for it.

Second Chakra Total = __________

Third Chakra: Solar Plexus

1. _______ I get overwhelmed by life's challenges.

2. _______ I have trouble bringing tasks to completion.

3. _______ I'm not sure what my purpose is.

4. _______ I feel intimidated by others.

5. _______ I struggle with low energy.

6. _______ I'm not very good at setting boundaries.

7. _______ My will gets distracted and goes in many directions.

Third Chakra Total = _________

Fourth Chakra: Heart

1. _______ I have trouble finding or maintaining intimate relationships.

2. _______ I am critical and judgmental of myself.

3. _______ I am critical and judgmental of others.

4. _______ I feel isolated and alone.

5. _______ I am shy about reaching out.

6. _______ Other people take too much energy from me.

7. _______ I hold a lot of grief in my heart.

Fourth Chakra Total = _________

Fifth Chakra: Throat

1. _______ I have trouble speaking what really matters to me.

2. _______ I tend to interrupt others when I should be listening.

3. _______ I have trouble getting my ideas across effectively.

4. _______ I wish I could be more creative.

5. _______ I often feel out of sync with others.

6. _______ I find it difficult to express myself in writing.

7. _______ Sometimes I don't know what's true in what people tell me.

Fifth Chakra Total = _________

Sixth Chakra: Third Eye

1. _______ I have trouble trusting my intuition.

2. _______ I have trouble imagining things different than they are.

3. _______ Sometimes I ignore that little voice inside.

4. _______ I rarely remember my dreams.

5. _______ I don't have a guiding vision for my life.

6. _______ I have trouble visualizing what I want.

7. _______ I don't really notice details around me.

Sixth Chakra Total = _________

Seventh Chakra: Crown

1. _______ I try to meditate but don't stick with it.

2. _______ I don't feel very connected to any kind of spirituality.

3. _______ I find it difficult to learn new things.

4. _______ I often think I'm just not smart enough.

5. _______ I am wary of new ideas.

6. _______ I'm not sure of my purpose.

7. _______ I don't know what I'm here for.

Seventh Chakra Total = _________

Scoring

All Chakras Total Score = _________

"Most of the time" in all columns (worst score) would be 5 x 49 = 245

"Never" in all columns (best score) would be 1 x 49 = 49

If you scored anything between about 100 and 245, it means there's room for improvement.

Chapter 4

MULADHARA CHAKRA
ROOT CHAKRA

Chakra 1	
Muladhar Chakra	English Name: Root Chakra
Mula Meaning	Root, Origin, Essence
Adhara Meaning	Basis, Foundation
Location	Perineum - Base of Spine. Coccyx, first 3 vertebrates at the base of the spine.
Element	Earth
Energy State	Solid
Purpose	Survival, grounding, Security, Stability, prosperity
Devil	Fear
Development	Womb to 12 months
Glands	Adrenal Glands (Fight – Flight)
Body parts	Legs, feet, bones, large Intestine, teeth
Malfunction	Obesity, anorexia, sciatica, constipation,hemorrhoids, degenerative arthritis, knee problems
Colour	Red. Our various mental states and emotions are related to specific Chakra color frequencies. Red is dense frequency.
Food	Protein
Rights	Right to be here, right to have

Understand our Root (Muladhara) Chakra

Let's begin from the beginning, with our scared ground, the ground we walk upon, our foundation. Just as strong tree needs strong roots, strong building needs a strong foundation, similarly we also need a solid base, a strong root which is grounded and stable. If you are going to build a bridge all the way to the heaven, its foundation needs to be really firm. This is our first chakra, the Muladhara Chakra, means root, support or foundation. The roots where we came from, the roots of our past, the roots of our beginnings. Anchored in the earth, that is the element of this chakra – **EARTH.**

Purpose of Root Chakra

The purpose of this chakra is to get grounded, to find stability, solidity and the ability to have things, to have security, to have trust, to have prosperity.

When we are born, we get delivered into our body, that's the vehicle in which we take our life's journey. We are given this body, so that we can achieve what we desire and create a materialistic life.

We only get one body per lifetime. So, it's really important to keep this vehicle in good shape.

Root Chakra Development

Chakras have different developmental stages in which the primary program of that chakra gets written into our mind-body interface or on our nervous system. And the development stage of this chakra is largely the first year of life.

When we are born the first challenge we have to face is to survive on our own. If we don't do that the game is over. So, first challenge is to survive and we are hardwired with instinct to survive.

Now when we are born, we are little, helpless bundle of protoplasm. We can't do much at all to ensure our own survival. We are dependent upon caretakers who feed us, who keeps us warm, who change our diapers, who keep us safe. And if that stage went well, we have a sense of trust that the world will provide what we need. That we are safe and we can relax and go on the life's journey.

What are we doing during our first year? We're building our body. The body weight triples during the first year of life. We're learning how things works, how do these fingers work? How do these toes work? How do I hold my head up? How do I keep food down and digest it? How do I deal with gravity and oh… that furniture has edges and that I can't go anywhere on my own? These are the kinds of things that consciousness of the body is trying to figure out. It's like getting a brand-new car and going okay where's the brakes, where's the peddles, where the gears. That's what we're trying to figure out in our body. And all of this time we're getting messages, **AM I SAFE?**

So, one of the first things that we establish in life is **trust versus mistrust.** Am I safe or am I not safe? Can I trust to take in from my environment in which I can nourish and grow or do I have to be careful? Do I have to check everything out?

Now when a child is this young, they don't have any language.

They don't have any preconceived notions; they just have raw experience. And through experiences, if they can't trust then what happens is everything contracts into the core. Imagine when you get fearful, you feel butterflies in your tummy area.

Constant sense of fear in child makes a very constricted core that doesn't have a lot of room for energy. What that does is it pushes all the energy up into the head away from the ground and out of first chakra.

So, this person might be very smart, always want to figure things out, but his nervous system doesn't feel safe to drop down, to rest, to expand and to open up and really fully have.

Chakra Blockages

So, we know that in this developmental stage we need to be safe, but what causes blockages?

- **Unsafe Environment:** This stage doesn't go well, if you don't feel safe, if your parents are busy or taking care of other children and you don't get fed when you're hungry. If there's violence in your surroundings. If its's noisy, if it's moving around a lot, your nervous system doesn't get to relax or get down. Well which direction is the ground? It's down. We say relax and let down. So, if want to relax we have to move down towards the earth.

- **Poor Mother Bonding:** If you didn't bond well with your mother, if there were feeding difficulties like a colicky baby who has trouble digesting and assimilating nourishment, then that can compromise the first chakra.

- **Feeling Unwanted:** If the child doesn't really feel like they belong here or they don't feel quite wanted. Maybe the mother doesn't want a baby or something in her nervous system was uncomfortable during pregnancy. The baby would have picked that up in the womb. And it might have given him a feeling of being unwanted. In this case the person will have to justify his existence, he will keep proving that he is worthy. In this case, we don't get to be in our natural organic state of just being and know that it's safe and easy to survive.

**That's why it is said that pregnant ladies need to be happy and stress free.

- **Horrendous birth processes:** The difficult birth processes traumatized child's nervous system. Generation that has traumatized nervous system will be disconnected from the earth.

So, when this stage doesn't go well, the natural result is FEAR. We learn Fear. You feel fearful when your survival is threatened. It's a natural feeling that actually should come up if somebody jumps out of a dark alley and points a gun at you, it's natural to feel that fear.

Your body floods with energy in order to run away or fight off your attacker (Fight or Flight response given by our adrenal gland).

But if a child gets that sense of fear because things don't feel quite right or they don't feel safe, that becomes a contraction in the body at the core level. And remember you're building your body at this stage. So, you build FEAR into the structure of the body until it becomes natural. Then you find that you are always worried, fearful and you can't relax even when you want to.

Our body is a set of habits and fear becomes a habit. Your body is constricted and you maybe grow very tall but very thin. Or you might compensate by putting on extra weight in order to feel safe. Fear becomes something we feel in our nervous system. When people have pervasive sense of fear in their body they look outside to say, what's wrong? Maybe that person isn't safe, maybe I need to do something, maybe I need to lock that door, maybe I need to double check that.

And that hyper-vigilance, it takes a lot of energy. It's like putting roadblocks up to what you can fully have.

Now of course we don't want to just be so trusting that we let anything in, we need adult reasonable discernment. But the habit of fear blocks you from receiving energy that you need to nourish yourself and your life.

Chakra Health and Balance

If you dealt with not feeling safe or wanted and you had survival concerns at young age, that's a wound in your first chakra. But you dealt with it in some way or another, by either creating excessive energy or deficient energy in the first chakra. **Chakras can be deficient, which results from an avoidant strategy, or excessive, resulting from a compensatory strategy.** In order to best function, each chakra needs to be balanced.

Excessive Energy in Root Chakra

If you have increased your energy to deal the devil of 1st Chakra i.e., Fear, then it looks like -

• Being overly attached to physical or materialistic things.

• May appear cynical about spiritual subjects, preferring the concrete proof.

• Over amping the survival instincts - Instinct to eat in order to live. That's why you eat too much. That's what your instinct is telling you and you fight with that your whole life.

Deficient Energy in Root Chakra

Or you could have gone to the deficient end of things. Deficient end wants to withdraw, wants to move out of the body. I don't want a big body, I don't want to weight much, I don't want to have lots of physical sense. I want to be up in my mind. I want to be up in the fantasy world. And often people who do that are very intelligent and very creative but

• They aren't very embodied. They are ungrounded

• They have a hard time getting over that sense of fear and distrust.

• Very thin body

• No interest in materialistic world

• Lives in scarcity

So, these are the ways the chakra can become unbalanced. But when you balance the chakras then you have a sense of trust in the world and trust in oneself. We cannot control the world outside to us, but we can surely control what inside us. Our reaction to things, our attitude towards life.

The survival instinct should be the base of our foundation and not the constant preoccupying issue.

Balanced Root Chakra

When our Muladhara Chakra is balanced we feel:

- More secure,

- More grounded,

- More stable,

- More confident and

- Freer to be who we truly are.

Exercise to understand your Root Chakra

Reflect on what you know about your birth experience and consider how it may be affecting you today (i.e., your sense of safety, security, worthy of having, and finances). If your parents are still alive, see what you can find out. Here are a few questions to start your reflection on (choose 3-4 questions that work for you. You do not have to answer all of them):

- Were you born in a hospital?

- Was your mother given medical drugs?

- Were there any complications? Were you in an incubator?

- How did this stage go for you in your earliest years? Were your survival needs provided?

- Did you have feeding difficulties? Were you bottle-fed or breast-fed?

- Did you feel safe in general growing up, even as you were an older child?

- Did you relax into your body? Did sleep in a crib?

- Did you bond well with your mother?

- Did you have to share this important period of bonding with other brothers and sisters?

Chapter 5

ROOT CHAKRA AND YOUR BUSINESS

Is your blocked Root Chakra sabotaging your Business Growth?

Our Root Chakra acts as the roots of a tree, grounding us into the Earth so our business can grow and expand. Now let's understand how our disbalanced root chakra affects our Business?

Your business is an extension of you. A disbalance in your root chakra also affects your business in some way or another.

When starting your business, you've got to hit the ground running (or be in the ground, grounding). You need to have a plan, a foundation, stability. Like roots in the ground, you need several avenues you can choose from. How grounded are you now?

In a nutshell, the Root Chakra of Business consists of:

• Our business plan (mission, values, vision, goals)

• Business model

• Organizational structures

• Systems processes and framework

- Standard operating procedures

- Clear customer avatar

- Solid offerings

- Financial stability

- Company culture

Let's have a look at what underlying issues are prevailing in your business, which is holding your growth and abundance.

How your Imbalanced Root Chakra affects your Business

- **Money Struggles** - Are you struggling with finances or money? Muladhara chakra is tied to our sense of security, it can make us feel safe or unsafe. It also has the ability to make us feel as though we live in abundance or scarcity, which means it is also tied to our quality of life and our financial situations. That's right, your root chakra has the ability to influence the amount of money you and your business is making.

- **Fear of failure** – The biggest devil of root chakra is fear. Fear of survival or fear of loss of our identity. Constant fear of failure doesn't let us take risks and challenges, which is a necessary ingredient of any business.

- **Unorganized** – You don't work with proper framework in mind, no documentation and you go around with lots of clutter in mind. This happens because you don't have clarity and grounding.

- **Afraid to sell** – Sales is an attitude. If your root chakra is disbalanced, you have the feeling of fear. Fear of not making the deal, or what people will say about you or your product/services. You shy away making upfront contact with your leads.

- **Feeling Stuck** – You feel stagnant in your business. You're not making progress as quickly as you'd like to or you're not sure which step to take next.

- **Easily angered.** You seem to have a short fuse —especially with those who you are closest to or work most closely with.

- **Excessive Anxiety or Worry** – You are plagued with worrisome thoughts of what might happen if. you lose a client, don't hit your revenue goals, fail, let your client down, get an unexpected bill, etc.

- You're experiencing **aches and pains** in your legs, feet or lower back or having issues with your colon or lower intestines.

- **Lack of trust** – Lack of trust on self-abilities, team, colleagues.

- **Lack Focus** – Difficult to focus at the task at hand. Get diverted easily and abandon tasks at slightest interruptions. Also leave task unfinished.

Balancing the Root Chakra

We are built for the nature. Yet we are sitting in front of the computers all day long, inside our office, A.C, travelling in train, buses, car etc. We are getting disconnected from the nature.

On a larger level we have

- Environmental Crisis

- Financial Crisis

- Health Crisis

All are root chakra issues on a larger scale.

When we fear, that keep people in scarcity, that makes them say to others - *oh you are my enemy, I have to keep as much as I want because you are going to take it away from me.*

We are living in this world that makes all of us less secure and less safe. It creates a culture of greed and mistrust.

If we are not living in abundance then there is something wrong with our relationship with the earth.

1. **Connect with nature:** It's essential to take time out of your busy schedule to foster a harmonious relationship with nature. Ever heard of the terms "earthing" or "grounding"? It's all about connecting with the Earth. Go outside and walk barefoot on the grass, dig your hands deep into the soil of your garden, take a few minutes to lay in the grass and soak up the rays of sunshine. Connecting with the earth element allows the root chakra to open and flow more freely.

2. **Plan nature retreats:** It resets your dials in the same way as

meditation does. Go out for vacation in nature to some nature Retreats. Get yourself disconnected from the technology for some days and feel the nature.

3. **Connect with your environment:** It's always important to connect with and feel stable in your own personal environment. Create spaces in your home and workplace that bring you joy and comfort. Develop a relationship with your community and its members. Be involved with as much as you feel necessary and attainable.

4. **Practise mindful eating:** Eating is our survival instinct, practise eating mindfully. Slow down, savour every bit. Choose food that are nourishing to you, so that you are nourishing your body and keeping it healthy.

5. **Have a positive mindset:** Instead of thinking what can go wrong, think what can go right. When you thinking from a positive angle, lots of opportunities start unfolding.

6. **Love yourself:** Start loving yourself. When you start loving yourself, you take care of yourself, you start loving and respecting others.

7. **Seed Mantra:** The mantra for Muladhara Chakra is LAM. Chanting the sanskrit word "LAM" vibrates from your vocal

cords all the way down to the tip of your spine, cleansing the root chakra of blockages that may be holding you back. Repeat this mantra during the day whenever you get time.

8. **Food:** Root vegetables are especially effective in balancing the root chakra because of their connection to the earth. Eat root vegetables like – beetroot, potatoes, sweet potatoes, carrot. Protein rich food like eggs, meats, beans, tofu, soy products, peanut butter is also good for giving energy to your body.

9. **Incorporate Red colour into your life:** Wear red clothes, decorate with the color red in your home or office. Red colour warms and revitalizes life force, courage and vitality.

10. **Carry grounding crystals with you:** Black tourmaline, Obsidian, Smokey Quartz, Hematite, Labradorite, Garnet, Ruby, Carnelian, Red Jasper and bloodstone are all very grounding and stabilizing stones to help you balance the energy in your root chakra.

11. **Burn candles or incense in earthy scents:** Like cedar wood, cloves, patchouli, musk, hyacinth or sandalwood.

12. **Meditate.** All forms of meditation are great but next time you meditate, try visualizing a clear, vibrant red light (like a protective bubble of energy) surrounding your body. Or, you can imagine that light as an energy sphere, the size of a grapefruit, at the base of your spine, swirling slowly and gracefully, calming and centring you.

13. **Create a strategic action plan.** Sit down and write out your goals for the year, breaking them down into achievable milestones and tasks that you can get started on right away. This will give you a clear sense of direction, prioritize tasks.

14. **Spend more time with the people who truly care about you.** Practice being authentic and vulnerable with the people you're closest to and ask for support when you need it. When you act like everything is okay (even when it's not) it can feel as if you're carrying the weight of the world on your shoulders all alone and nobody cares about you. But really, they just don't know you are in need of support. When you open up to others and give them the chance to support you, they will. And you'll start to feel more supported, loved and cared for than ever.

15. If money is a source of anxiety for you, take the time to educate yourself and **create a financial plan** that will ease the stress and give you the sense of security you need. This may involve developing a budget, paying off debt, reducing expenses, increasing marketing efforts or creating multiple revenue streams, hiring a team, selling assets, etc. Once you've developed your financial plan, start taking action to move yourself toward your goals. The act of making progress will give you a sense of accomplishment and help to ease the anxiety by putting you back in control and giving you a sense of security in knowing you're on track to make your financial dreams a reality.

16. Affirmations: Quit making yourself wrong and approach yourself with compassion. You want to go back to the ground and you want to tell yourself I am welcome here. You want to welcome yourself into your own body. Pick some affirmations and keep reminding yourself with the statements.

- It is safe for me to be here.

- I love my body and trust its wisdom

- I am IN here.

- The earth supports me.

- I live in abundance.

- I hold my ground no matter what I encounter.

Chapter 6

SVADHISTHANA CHAKRA
SACRAL CHAKRA

Chakra 2	
Svadhisthana Chakra	English Name: Sacral Chakra
Svadhisthana Meaning	One's own place
Location	Lower abdomen 3 inches below navel. Sacrum, Lumbar spine, lower abdomen.
Elementww	Water
Energy State	Liquid
Purpose	Desire, pleasure, sexuality, feeling, emotions
Devil	Guilt
Development	6 months to 2 years
Glands	Reproductive, Sex Glands
Body parts	Pelvis, genitals, reproductive system, kidney, bladder, lower back
Malfunction	In the body, the sacral chakra connects with reproductive parts. Issues like (infertility, impotence, or menstrual issues) and lower back, kidney, or stomach disorders are effects of malfunction in this chakra
Colour	Orange
Food	Liquid
Rights	To feel

Understand our Sacral (Svadhisthana) Chakra

Let's take the next step into our second chakra, the sacral chakra. Here we move from earth to water, from self to others, from one to two, unity to duality. It's a big step with big changes. Let's dive into it.

The purpose of each chakra is to be able to bridge the link from earth till heaven. As discussed in previous chapter the purpose of our 1st chakra is to get grounded and stable in making a foundation. Once the foundation is built, we move to the upper chakras and the next in line is our Svadhisthana chakra. The purpose of the second chakra is to get things moving, to have a flow.

The element of the second chakra is water, whose property is flow, movement. Water flows the path of least resistance; it takes the shape of earth.

So, we want to flow, we want to be full and juicy. When things are dry, they don't have enough water, they are no fun.

If you want your life to be juicy, open this chakra and bring water element into it.

Purpose of this Chakra

The main purpose of this chakra is to feel, to move energy and to increase your capacity for pleasure, to enjoy life to the fullest. Feeling is an important aspect of our consciousness. We get the feedback from the environment in terms of our feelings. Are we on the right track? Are we on the wrong track? Does it feel good? Does it feel bad?

When we feel pain, it's a message that we need some kind of change to do something different. Feeling is an important navigator that we can use wisely to access our life's journey.

Chakra Development

After we have learned how to operate our body mainly through the 1st year, there is an overlap with the 2nd chakra mainly around 6 months. This chakra come into play once movement is possible for the child, which is around 6 months.

What happens to the six months old?

The eyes change its ability to focus. Instead of just being right in front of the face like staring at the mother's face when she is holding baby in her arms, the child is now able to focus across the room. So, we start sitting up and we see across the room.

And what do you think is created in the child's psyche?

Curiosity

The desire to see what is over there. And that curiosity makes the child move. So the next development that happens is Creeping-Crawling-Walking-Running. Once you learn to move by your own, you get busy exploring the things around you.

You explore through your senses. Eyes, Ears, Touch, Taste, Smell. Senses are the gateway which brings the outside world to us. And while learning about the world they are developing an awareness about the things. Is it safe or not safe? Is it good or bad? When I touch a hot stove, we get hurt, it's not good to touch it. When mummy gives an ice cream, it tastes pretty good, I want to eat that again.

We create awareness about what is pleasurable and what is painful. We all want to move away from painful and move towards pleasurable experiences.

We develop emotional literacy at this stage. Good, bad, happy, sad, angry. We start to identify our feelings. And later on, start expressing our feelings appropriately.

We develop an emotional connect with our caretakers. That's something we feel

- We feel good in mother's or father's arms

- We feel good in our own home. More than feeling safe, the emotions come into picture and we start feeling good, pleasurable. The pleasure of being alive.

Small kids don't know the language yet. So, if they get hurt, they cry. That's an emotional communication for the child that something is wrong. If parent or caretaker respond to their emotional needs, they take them from pain to pleasure, then their nervous system gets relaxed, limbic system says everything is alright and the child feel good again.

Chakra Blockages

The blockages in this chakra develops because of any of the following reasons:

- **Denial of child's feeling state:** Not listening or understanding what kid wants to say or express. Ignoring the kid with statements like - You are not right to feel that way. Stop here or you are so sensitive or you cry all the time. Then our feeling state is denied and we are knocked out of our own place.

- **Unpleasant or painful environment:** When there is lot of anger, violence in the environment, we restrict our movement of flow

- **Kid also learns to speak the emotional language of the family:** If your family was not very expressive, you also learn not to express your feelings.

Chakra Health and Balance

The name of this chakra is Svadhisthana which means one's own place. The challenge of this chakra is to be connected to your own self inside. That is a feeling state, where we feel comfortable in our own skin. When we feel comfortable, then energy flows.

But when our emotions and feelings are restricted, we get out of touch with our own self, and we lose touch with others. We become numb towards how we feel for ourselves or for others.

This is what is happening in our society, we are told to deny pleasure, emotions, feelings, doing something good for ourselves or even thinking about self is not good. It's a sign of weakness to show our emotions. Statement like boys don't cry or girls can't be violent conditions us to hide our emotions. Emotions are a natural process, which will erupt, but if we deny or hide it every time, we get numb to our feelings, then we need sensationalism to open our numbness and we do bad things to self and to each other. Rape, violence, addictions are increasing today, because we are out of touch with ourselves.

We don't even know what we feel anymore. What happens we become out of touch? We do things that don't feel good to ourselves and to others and planet. We are misled into doing wrong things and then we don't feel the effects.

We also numb our feelings in terms of sexuality. This chakra is located where we human beings have their reproductive organs, ovary in women and testosterones in male. Sexualism is a natural body process. It helps to share the emotions and feelings with each other. In today's world sexualism is both supressed and then sensationalism. We are told that its wrong or bad, and then it's used in all sorts of advertising, movies etc. We are out of balance in this chakra. And if you look at the world, we have flood and droughts. The water element is totally out of balance. When water is damned it erodes the stream banks. So, we need to free up this flow but in an appropriate manner, with appropriate boundaries, appropriate containment. There was research that the cultures that supress emotions and sexuality, shows and increase in violence. And the culture that are open, and take care of feelings and emotions shows a decrease in violence.

Our emotions become unbalanced. The charge of our emotions become unbalanced and this chakra becomes unbalanced.

Excessive Sacral Chakra

We may develop excessive charge in this chakra. Which means too much water.

- Over indulge in order to compensate for the pleasurable life. We may eat that cookie or we may have that drink.

- Over indulge in fantasies, sexual obsession.

- Over emotional. Some people only feel alive only when they are having intense emotions.

Deficient Sacral Chakra

Or we may have deficient chakra which is an avoidance response, which is categorise as

- Flat emotionally. Become numb to any feeling or emotions.

- Feels that life is dull and boring. It's not fun and juicy anymore.

- Lack sexual desires and satisfaction

- Stuck in a particular feeling for long.

People always ask me can I have excess and deficient chakra at the same time. I say yes, and especially in this chakra which involves both emotions and sexuality. Some people are highly sexual and not very emotional while some are highly emotional and not very sexual.

One more thing that we develop in the chakra is the feeling of GUILT. We feel guilty about the way we feel. I shouldn't be feeling this way about this person or I shouldn't want this or I shouldn't need that, we feel guilty about doing something good for ourselves, thinking about us first or praising us. And guilt stops the flow of energy. Now if you have done something and hurt somebody's feelings then it's appropriate to feel this way and to apologise and make amends. But if GUILT becomes a normal norm for you then that you have to correct it.

For example, when I spend more time on myself, like exercise or meditation I feel guilty that I should be spending more time at work, and when I spend more time at work, I feel guilty of not spending enough time with my kid. So that Guilt feeling keeps popping up. So, one day I said to myself, enough is enough, I cannot keep thinking this way all the time. I need to prioritize things and choose things. What do I want?

This feeling of guilt hinders the natural flow of emotions and desires.

Once you master this feeling of overcoming you guilt you

• Can truly enjoy your life. You will enjoy all the wonders of life like your meal, sunset, sunrise, sexuality. It's not about doing anything we want without thinking and feeling guilty, that of course would be over indulgence. We want to have appropriate feeling in the body.

• You harvest the gift of extreme pleasure

• Maintains healthy sexual and emotional boundaries

When we block the flow of feelings, we become rigid. The roots won't grow until we water them. When we restrict the feelings the movement of the energy wont flow through the body. To move from solid to liquid, what do we do, we melt. So, as we melt our rigidity, we melt our fixed patterns and come into the flow. We have a river of energy inside us, that can flow and nurture any part of the body.

Let's move the flow of water and change the world.

Exercise

To reclaim your right to feel deeper, first gain awareness and acknowledge where you got lost in the first place? Reflect and answer:

- What were you taught about your feelings in your family? Were you allowed to feel and express your emotions? Was there any support?

- What feelings have remained unexpressed?

- What did you need as a child that you didn't get?

- What did you get that you didn't want?

- What did you do as a result of not getting your needs met?

- How does that affect your ability to recognize and meet your needs now?

- How does that affect your emotional boundaries with yourself and others?

*There may be a lot coming up for you. Don't feel the need to understand everything all at once. Be the observer of your own process. This is the beginning of a new awareness, which is the first step in the journey.

....

....

....

....

....

....

....

....

....

....

Chapter 7

SACRAL CHAKRA AND YOUR BUSINESS

Is your blocked Sacral Chakra sabotaging your Business Growth?

As discussed in the previous chapter our svadhisthana chakra is the creative centre of the body. It connotes all things joyous, and beautiful and creative. Just like your brand is the creative part of your business that carries the rest of your processes through. Without a good brand, you won't be able to get very far in business. A strong brand is a strong business. And if you're just starting off, have fun with this, keep your brand balanced and consistent by doing your research on color psychology.

In nutshell the Sacral Chakra of your business is related to:

• Brand positioning

• Brand image

• Brand consistency

• Social media

• Content production

• Creative works

- Brand awareness

- Company morale

How your imbalanced Sacral Chakra affects your Business

- **Afraid of Marketing:** You think it's a difficult process, because either you don't know the right process or you are afraid of what people might say. Marketing is vital for any business and if you are shying away from marketing, then you are up for a big trouble.

- **Don't have a defined Brand:** How you define your brand and what it means to your business can help guide both your brand and business forward. With alignment around is what makes your brand unique, you can build a marketing strategy around it and allow your brand to reach its full potential.

- **Lack inspiration:** This can be the biggest hurdle for you to reach to your goals. Lack of motivation cripples you to take any action.

- **Fuzzy creative directions:** Sacral Chakra is our creative chakra. It waters the creativity inside us. If sacral chakra is blocked then you are not able to wear your creative hat.

- **Unclear Business vision:** Of all the reasons responsible for why you might be lacking in the motivation department, this one is by far the most common: Either you don't know what you want, or there's a lack of clarity about what you want. This leads to unclear business vision.

- **Struggle to create connections:** You feel numb and disconnected with your team and people around. When your emotional chakra is blocked, your lack social skills and avoid people as far as possible.

- **Losing your passion and enthusiasm into your business:** You starts enthusiastically, but gradually your passion starts depleting. You lack inspiration, to do any task and doing any activity looks monotonous. Your business and its operations don't seem fun and pleasurable to you anymore.

If these are the issues, that's a sign that your sacral chakra is blocked and needs attention.

How to Balance Svadhisthana Chakra

1. **Get creative:** Engage in some creative activity like painting, poetry, writing books, blogs. When we were kids, we had hobbies, but growing up where did it go. Do you still have a hobby, something which you do where you forget your time? Consider this essential for the growth of ourself and your company.

2. **Reclaim your feelings:** Share your feelings with each other. There is a power in sharing. Because our feelings want to be

witnessed, they want to be understood. Sometimes they are there until we share them. When someone says, "I understand what you are feeling", and we go ah I don't have to carry this anymore. It's a way of making deeper connection. Some people are excessive, and they spill their emotions all over. These people should learn to contain. They need to learn that I don't have to dump my anger on this person, I don't have to cry until I am exhausted. Take charge of your body. Others who are too emotionally flat, they need to learn to open up, to express it to other people. So, you probably know whether you fall in the excessive side or deficient side and whether you need to open up or contain.

3. **Stop and notice what you feel:** Allow the emotion to surface and try to understand the information they are trying to surface. We all are human being, we all have emotions, we all are on the same boat floating on the sea. There are no good or bad emotions. We don't choose how we feel, we choose what we do about those feelings. Feelings come up on their own.

4. **Maintain a journal:** Have a conversation with your thoughts and feelings. Sometimes our emotions need attention and writing in on the paper of how you feel gives due attention to them. I conduct morning sessions with Entrepreneur where we all write about our thoughts and emotions without any filtrations. This way we clear our headspace and can focus on our goals. Write to me (coach.manika@gmail.com to know more about the Entrepreneur Success Morning Rituals).

5. **Don't be Judgemental:** Pull back the judgement of ourselves and others. Most of us have harsh inner critics who judge us, put us down, and punish us when we make mistakes. As long as you have an inner general beating you up for your inevitable imperfections, you'll find it difficult to create connections with self and others. What if we could just let go of all the dualistic judgments that label everything as "right" or "wrong," "good" or "bad?" What if, instead, we could just trust that life is hard and everyone is doing the best they can? Releasing judgment of others starts with letting go of self-judgments.

6. **Practise compassion:** When you commit to practicing compassion, your relationships become more intimate. Negative feelings will start to lessen. Your mind becomes quieter, allowing you to receive clearer inner guidance. You become more attractive to people you meet because they can feel your heart.

7. **Water Therapy:** The element of sacral chakra is water. Immerse yourself in water to relax yourself when feeling low emotionally. Keep yourself well hydrated. Water has healing power. Taking a quick bath or splashing your face with water is a quick remedy to uplift your mood and relaxing you.

8. **Mediation Music:** Listen to any kind of flowing water music meditation to relax you down. A lot of these are available on youtube.

9. Seed Mantra: Chant the seed mantra "VAM" every day.

10. Branding: Work with some professional agency to create your company's logo and marketing material. This is essential, don't skip this part.

11. Mission and Vision: Define proper mission and vision of the company, which keeps you on track and pumps the enthusiasm continuously.

12. Network: Join some community or networking group of like-minded people which helps you to in your business and personal growth.

13. Corporate Social Responsibility (CSR): Do some social service act as a part of mandatory business requirement. That will help you in building compassion towards others.

14. Gemstones: Wearing gemstones like coral,carnelian,yellow zircon open up your emotional richness.

15. Colour: Orange is the colour of sacral chakra. Orange colour stimulates, encourages and renews energy and frees you from rigid emotional pattern.

16. Affirmations: Repeat the affirmations listed below.

- I deserve pleasure
- I feel good.
- I embrace and celebrate my sexuality.
- It is safe to feel my emotions.
- I listen to my feelings.
- Life is pleasurable.

Chapter 8

MANIPURA CHAKRA
SOLAR PLEXUS CHAKRA

Chakra 3	
Manipura Chakra	English Name: Solar Plexus Chakra
Manipura Meaning	Lustrous Gem
Location	Above your navel and below your sternum, in the solar plexus area
Element	Fire
Energy State	Plasma
Purpose	Will, power, energy
Devil	Shame
Development	18 months to 3 years
Glands	It is related to energy, assimilation and digestion, and is said to correspond to the roles played by the pancreas and the outer adrenal glands, the adrenal cortex. These play a valuable role in digestion, the conversion of food matter into energy for the body.
Body parts	Digestive system, liver, gall bladder
Malfunction	Digestives troubles, chronic fatigue, hypertension.
Colour	Yellow
Food	Starches
Rights	To Act

Understand our Solar Plexus (Manipura) Chakra

Welcome to solar plexus our 3rd chakra whose element is fire. We started from earth, build our foundation, moved to water, got fluid and flowing, where the energy started to move. And now we will take fire and movement and create energy. Take your hands, rub them together, your hand is matter, rubbing them is movement, feel how it creates heat or energy. That's how this chakra is build.

Purpose of this Chakra

Our purpose is to find our power, to develop the strength of our will, to develop strength in our bodies, to increase the amount of energy we have and to be able to really direct that energy into the activities of our choice. That's following through on our will.

Why is this important? If we didn't have our will in place, nothing would ever change. There would be no evolution. We will still be in the first or second chakra, that is subject to gravity, water will find its path of least resistance. It will go wherever it wants to. But we need our will to go in a new direction. We need our will to do the work of our choice. We need our will to say that I will not eat junk food and direct my energies in building a healthy and energetic body. You need to have your power in order to make change.

Chakra Development

The developmental stage of this chakra is approximately 18

months to 3-4 years. So, what's happening at this time? A child has gone through the second chakra of exploring the world around and they have been developing language. As they started to move, to explore their environment, their parents tell them what to do like don't touch that, don't do that, be quiet, hold still, hold back. Through this the child learns impulse control. This is essential to learn before we can socialize in the next chakra. But how this goes depends how the child is taught. Is the child being overly controlled or they have the freedom to express themselves. The child is learning to move out from the symbiosis of his parents, so at this stage the child is developing their autonomy and their will. They are saying, no I don't want to do that, and they are learning to tie their shoes, or to button their shirts, hold up a cup and eat right, and they are learning how to do things. This is actually the development of the ego identity and self-definition.

At this stage the development of following happens:

• Development of autonomy

• Will

• Self esteem

• Impulse control

And the way we are taught gets coded in our subconscious programming.

Do we have a sense of power that we can control our circumstances to a certain degree or not? Do we take charge of the situation? Do we complete the task? Do we handle what life gives us or not? Are we safe to challenge authority? Are we safe to go in a new direction? Do you remain true to your own purpose, or do you even have a sense of purpose?

These are all the aspects that we develop in the third chakra.

Chakra Blockages

- **Shame** – As we are learning to take action, and someone says, oh, you did that so well. We get a feeling of pride; we get a feeling of self-esteem. And if we are shamed for doing a task, oh you don't know how to do it right, we lose our confidence. We start to equate our doing and accomplishing the task as who we are. And if we don't do well, we think we are bad.

- **Authoritative parents** – Who doesn't allow kid to have his or her own will

- **Age-Inappropriate responsibilities** – When a young child has to take care of his younger siblings, it's a responsibility that can leave a child feeling inadequate, because the child doesn't know that he is not old enough to do that. If it is expected of them, they start expecting it of themselves.

- **Over protective parents** – Doesn't allow kids to search his own path.

- **Not being allowed to be different** – "You will have to do this only. You got to do what everybody in the family does", some phrases that can hamper the child's individuality.

Chakra Health and Balance
Deficient

- Weak Will – We don't follow on things

- We hold back our power – Not standing for ourselves or others

- Not take charge of the situation - It can make us passive or passive aggressive, where we pretend not to be rebelling against something, but we are in a passive way.

- Low confidence

- Low energy

Excessive

- Over-controlling

- Dominating - When you grow in powerlessness situation, that creates love for power. You grow up and say I don't want to be dominated. And then we do just like everybody else, we dominate, because that what we have been taught that power means dominance.

- Aggressive

- Powerful and always in a fight mode.

- Excessively doing – doing something all the time, over active. In the long run that could lead to exhaustion.

The imbalances led us to be afraid to own our power and then we become victim of our own circumstances, instead of being the creators of the life we want. We fall into resentment and resentment leads to resistance, and resistance is like driving a car with the brakes on. We are doing what we are told, we don't really want to do it, so we drag ourselves. Many a times people resist even things that they are choosing for themselves. This creates wastage of your energy. The energy which should have been put to create a life you want, your life's mission and purpose. We need energy to come into power.

If you were shamed, you lost your power. You might have that inner critic that voice at the back of your head telling you, you are not good. You might have feelings of worthlessness. This vicious inner critic is like the anger that should have come out to take charge of your life, hits the wall and turns back against the self.

You might self-sabotage, we think that we won't succeed, then why even try. We blame others for all the troubles in our life. That's a sure sign that you are giving away your power.

Shame comes from outside and when we overcome that we have

• Energy

• Strong will and effective action

• Sense of personal power – We live in a faulty meaning of power. We think that power is having absolute control. Its dominating other people, but that disempowers us. What is empowering someone is disempowering other. That creates disbalance in the world. Real power comes when we put things together.

If the chakra is balanced, then you are

• **Proactive**. You think and do your task ahead of time. You plan things properly to take the outcome you want.

• Responsible and Reliable

• Effective Will

• Confident

Exercise

Reflect and explore these questions:

- Who held power in your family household?

- What means did they use to establish their authority? (Punishment, dominance, emotional manipulation, etc.)

- How did you react at the time? (Comply, rebel, withdraw, manipulate, or something else?)

- What do you do now? (Do you still tend to comply, rebel, etc.?) What form does the inner authority take in your life now?

- Become aware of more choices in how to respond (negotiate, communicate, collaborate, win/win).

- If you had your power back from wherever you lost it, what would you do with it now? Is there any situation where you're repeating the same pattern of response? Take responsibility for your part. Choose another response. Power only exists when it is being applied.

SOLAR PLEXUS AND YOUR BUSINESS

Is your blocked Solar Plexus sabotaging your Business growth?

It takes strength, confidence, determination, and will power to put yourself out there. That's what the solar plexus and marketing have in common. When you have a balanced Solar plexus chakra, these attributes shine through you like the sun. Marketing is much the same. It takes these traits to become successful, to keep going after the countless **NO's,** to have will power and determination to hear that **YES.** However, an unbalanced solar plexus can turn into unethical and unhealthy business practice. When a solar plexus is out of balance, one becomes controlling, competitive, power hungry, or the opposite and feels powerless. One or the other is not good in your body or in business. Know that you have the power to succeed!

The solar plexus of business consists of:

- Leadership skill

- Rules and regulations

- Management

- Powerful messaging

- Confidence in your work

- Customer psychology

- Conversion

- Selling

- Affiliates

How your imbalanced Solar Plexus Chakra affects your Business

- **Spend lot of time comparing yourself and your business with others:** This behaviour crops from low self-esteem. We don't know or devalue our own worth. This gives you a strong competition anxiety and fear of failure.

- **Suffer from Low energy most of the time:** Feeling tired and lethargic on a regular basis is extremely common symptom of blocked chakra. This chakra is related to energy, assimilation and digestion. These play a valuable role in digestion, the conversion of food matter into energy for the body. If this chakra doesn't function properly, the body and mind doesn't get sufficient fuel to take action.

- **Difficult for you to focus:** The fire element inside you is undirected. You sit for a task but unable to concentrate. The vital energy flow is blocked off and this can result in feelings of physical, mental and emotional exhaustion.

- **Suffer from a disease called as Procrastination:** If one of your inner belief systems or thought patterns is, I am unworthy, then one of the outer effects will probably be procrastination. After all, procrastination is one way to keep us from getting where we say we want to go. Most people who procrastinate will spend a lot of time and energy berating themselves for procrastination. They will call themselves lazy and generally will make themselves out to feel they are bad person. Do you wait for the last moment to complete the task and miss deadlines most of the time?

- **Most of the time you don't show up to meetings and events:** The solar plexus chakra governs your self-image, expression, and acceptance of your authentic personality. When this chakra is blocked you will probably experience a feeling of loss of identity. You will feel disconnected from yourself and shy away from others.

- **Weak will:** You think too much but shy away to take action. If you have an underactive solar plexus chakra you are more likely to be pulled into energy-draining and overwhelming emotional states such as helplessness and shame. This pulls you back from taking action.

- **Blame others, competitors, environment, government etc for your troubles and losses:** When the solar plexus chakra is unbalanced this can result in feeling and experiencing being easily taken advantage of. You may have an inferiority complex that makes you feel like you don't deserve, don't belong, and that you are the victim of your life situation. Because this chakra is the energy center of confidence, self-awareness, self-acceptance, and personal power when you are unbalanced in this chakra it can manifest as a victimhood mentality.

If yes, then your 3rd Chakra, needs attention.

How to Balance Manipura Chakra

1. Live with Integrity: We have to live with Integrity. Define your values and live by what really important to you. I have listed some of the core values to take reference and inspiration. Define your own core value and live by it. Once you define your values put your actions with your value system.

Authenticity	**Fame**	**Peace**
• Achievement	• Friendships	• Pleasure
• Adventure	• Fun	• Poise
• Authority	• Growth	• Popularity
• Autonomy	• Happiness	• Recognition
• Balance	• Honesty	• Religion
• Beauty	• Humor	• Reputation
• Boldness	• Influence	• Respect
• Compassion	• Inner Harmony	• Responsibility
• Challenge	• Justice	• Security
• Citizenship	• Kindness	• Self-Respect
• Community	• Knowledge	• Service
• Competence	• Leadership	• Spirituality
• Contribution	• Learning	• Stability
• Creativity	• Love	• Success
• Curiosity	• Loyalty	• Status
• Determination	• Meaningful Work	• Trustworthiness
• Fairness	• Openness	• Wealth
• Faith	• Optimism	

2. **Take RISK:** Take a chance. See what happens. It may not be as bad as you think it is. You may be able to set up and as you do you will be able to fly.

3. **Increase your confidence:** You can increase your skill by doing some courses, suiting your requirement.

4. **Be proactive:** Plan your time and task well before time. Make it a habit of listing down your task first thing in the morning, and then go on accomplishing it one by one.

5. **Learn and develop leadership skills:** There are several core leadership skills that are considered important traits to help you become a more effective leader. Whether it's taking the initiative, developing critical thinking skills, or learning how to motivate and empower those around you, you must constantly be challenging yourself to enhance your leadership capabilities.

6. **Journal:** Maintain journal of all the good achievements of yours. This increases self-esteem. Give gratitude to yourself – your body, mind, challenges that you have overcome, your abilities etc. We all have some qualities which makes us who we are. List down all your qualities and traits.

7. **Believe in yourself:** Trust yourself that you can do it. Start believing in yourself. Be kind to yourself. Begin to love and approve of yourself.

8. **Define your Goals:** Write down your personal and professional goals to gain more clarity in your actions.

9. **Business Model Clarity:** Define a well-structured funnel model of your business to know in which direction you have to take action.

10. **Psychotherapy sessions:** Take psychotherapy sessions like ego building, release anger, work on shame issues, strengthen the will. This will help to rebuild you.

11. **Expose yourself to Sunlight:** Take sunlight in the morning. Its good for our health both physically and mentally.

12. **Own your will:** Whatever you are doing, whether you want to do it or not, you are doing with your will. Reframe blaming

others for your circumstances. Take charge of your life and situation. Look at this way, if it's their fault, there's nothing you can do about it. But if you take charge of the situation, you are empowering yourself to change it.

13. **Choose your words:** Instead of saying "I have to" say "I choose to. I choose to pay my bills, because I want to keep the lights on. I choose to do this and that will empower your will. Cause when we say I have to automatically has resistance coming in, "yeah I have to but I don't want to".

14. **Reclaim your Power:** We live in a faulty meaning of power. We think that power is having absolute control. Its dominating other people, owing more money. That disempowers us. What is empowering someone is disempowering others. That creates disbalance in the world. Real power comes when we put things together. We join together, we cooperate, collaborate and work together.

15. **Gemstones:** Wearing gemstones like Tiger's eye, Amber, Topaz, Citrine brings balance, warmth and confidence.

16. **Seed Mantra:** Chant the seed mantra "RAM" every day.

17. **Colour:** Yellow colour or golden hue compensates inner fatigue, creates joy and promotes relaxation.

18. Affirmations

- I honour the power within me.
- I follow through with my will.
- My inner fire burns through blocks and fears.
- My will and divine will are aligned.
- I know my purpose.
- I accomplish easily and effortlessly.

Chapter 10

ANAHATA CHAKRA
HEART CHAKRA

Chakra 4	
Anahata Chakra	English Name: Heart Chakra
Anahata Meaning	Unstruck
Location	Heart
Element	Air
Energy State	Gas
Purpose	Love, peace, compassion
Devil	Grief
Development	3.5 years to 7 years
Glands	Thymus Gland
Body parts	Lungs, heart, circulatory system, arms, hands
Malfunction	Asthama, coronary disease, lung disease
Colour	Green
Food	Vegetables
Rights	To Love

Understanding our Heart (Anahata) Chakra

Now we have reached to the Heart chakra. Let's understand the heart chakra, how to balance this chakra whose element is air and fly in our life to its full potentiality.

It's an integrator between Lower chakras which are more practical chakra and upper chakras which are spiritual chakras.

Purpose of Heart Chakra

Purpose of heart chakra is to expand beyond ourselves. The below three chakras is about ourselves, which is important because first we need to know who we are. But the upper four chakras get beyond our ego. Heart chakra is about love, about connection, about relationship, compassion, forgiveness, acceptance, generosity and the peace that comes from balance.

Chakra Development

We enter the heart chakra around 4 years old up to 7 years, where we are integrating into the social world. After we get the impulse control in 3rd chakra, we are ready to socialize. We are toilet trained, we know when to be quiet, we can control our actions and not hit somebody, we learn to greet people. Now we are ready to go to kinder garden school, we are ready to play with our younger or elder brother or sister, or kids of the neighbourhood. Every child from the moment they are born wants to be loved. But until we have impulse control it's not much we can do about it. But once we develop that mind over matter, we can control ourselves in a way that we can think can bring love.

So, if your mother likes it when you are really quiet, you don't ask anything, then maybe you learn that's how you will get love and you do that lifelong, being quite to get love. Or maybe being helpful or being funny at school or good at sports or really smart brings you approval. And as we get the feedback from our surroundings of what people like and don't like we start to develop our personality. The word personality comes from the word persona that means mask.

We get this programming from our school, from television, from parents, brothers and sisters. We develop these personalities to go out into the world. But sometimes it's different from our authentic self.

We learned that our vulnerability is not safe or we learned that we can't show that we don't know something. In this case our authentic self gets buried and we start living in that persona which everybody sees and like or we think they like.

Carrying a particular persona is fine when you are in a work place or out on the street, but you don't want to be carrying your persona every time in your relationship or your personal space. We want relationship to be connected with our authentic selves.

If we are not in our authentic self, we don't trust that love is real. We think that the other person loves me because I am smart or intelligent or good looking or I make money etc. Instead of who I really am. And we're all longing to have that deep connection, to be understood and most of all to be loved.

Chakra Blockages

Love is important in our childhood and well as adulthood. We are human beings we need love in all the stages of our lives.

• Rejection, abandonment, loss of loved ones like parents, divorce or even moving around (transfers) and losing a friend. In this case a child has to start all over again, making a friend in a new school. We stop trusting that we can have an open heart and can keep connections with people.

• Many children are raised with conditional love that is, go to your room and come down when you can be nice or you can smile. Then we relate that we can get love only if we do certain things. This splits us from the authentic self.

• If you had a very critical parent. You have internalized that critical voice. And on the other hand, if you had a loving parent then that got internalize in your system and you know how to be good to yourself and others. One important thing about self-love is that it is conditioned by the relationship we have, especially with our parents. They become internalized.

• Child abuse (emotional and physical).

Child gets a confusing message that maybe punishment means love, or controlling means love, dominating means love. All this is conditioned into the system of the child and that carries through the adult relationship looking for that authentic love.

So as a consequence, we learn not to trust love, and some of it shows up as being judgemental or isolated, having a closed heart where you won't really let people in or being afraid to be vulnerable or maybe not asking for help because you think its selfish. At a later stage because of this you avoid intimate relationship.

If everyone would have been perfect then there would be no need for love. No one is perfect yet we love our friends, family and accept them with their imperfection and vulnerability, because we like them who they are, similarly they like and accept us for who we are. And that goes for especially for loving ourself.

Chakra Health and Balance

As a parent is to the child so is the mind to the body. If your parents abandon you, you will abandon yourself, if your parents mistreated you, you will mistreat yourself. If your parents respected you, you will respect yourself.

Excessive

- Co-dependent – I am more in everybody else's business, than I am in mine

- Poor Boundaries in a relationship

- Abuser or abused in relationships

- Jealousy

- Possessive

- Demanding
- Needs to be the centre of attention at all the time.

Deficient

- Anti – social
- Doesn't trust love
- Cold or intolerant or critical
- Not compassionate

Balance

- Compassionate
- Loving
- Empathetic
- Feeling for others and self
- Self-loving
- We just go around with an open heart

Exercise

Answer deeper questions in the workbook like.

- List things that you like about yourself
- Name something you don't like about yourself
- Look back in your life and see when that trait began. How old were you? 5 years, 7 years.

- Forgive yourself in those places that you typically judge. And make a space in your heart.

Chapter 11

HEART CHAKRA AND YOUR BUSINESS

Is your blocked Heart Chakra sabotaging your business?

We human beings are social animals. We need love, need relationships, we make connections. The heart of a business is the people that come into your life, or walk through the door! And because of the people, our lives and businesses can thrive.

When someone has a balanced heart Chakra, they are able to give and receive love well and without constraint. In business this may appear in the form of a smooth transaction, where you are willing to receive a payment with enthusiasm, and eager to render your services to do the best work you can in return.

In Business this chakra relates to:

• Community Building

• Connection to your audience

• Customer service

• Testimonials

• Referrals

• Giving and receiving

• Emotional satisfaction of your employees

How blocked Heart Chakra affects your business?

• **Afraid to sell:** Selling is basically making connections with your target audience. You are afraid of selling because you are not comfortable with or around people. You fear rejection, criticism, or judgement by people.

• **You feel like you are giving too much value of the price you are getting:** Do you believe that you don't have control over your product/services price? It is dictated by the market, where you have to give more value and in return the price is not sufficient?

• **Trust issues with your employees, colleagues or your partners:** When heart is heavy or closed it becomes difficult to trust people. This makes it difficult to delegate any task. And since running a successful business is a team work, the end result is the growth of business hampers.

• **Feel like giving up:** You are lost on your mission, because of your inability to make connections inside and outside your business. The motivation and inspiration with which you started your business starts dying down as the required results doesn't come up and you feel heavy or broken.

- **Nervous to invest in yourself and your growth:** Heart chakra is about loving self as well. When you don't see yourself valuable, you hesitate to take steps for your self-growth.

- **You feel like you are working in the business and not on it:** You're not using your Genius, that means you're stuck in day to day operations and probably don't feel connected to what you do. This is because you are unable to delegate the basic operational work to your team or you are not able to hire the right people. Instead of you strategizing about the company's growth you are spending time on daily operational work, which can be easily delegated. Remember "Busyness is not Business".

- **Lack compassion:** You are critical and judgemental about yours and others actions. It's difficult for you to forget and forgive people for their mistakes. You are closed when needed by someone and becomes defensive when challenged.

How to balance your Heart Chakra

1. **Lighten your Heart:** The demon of heart chakra is GRIEF. And grief is a natural response to losing someone you love. Grief is heavy like a stone and the element of heart is light. So, when we have too much grief there's a heaviness inside. You have to work through your grief to shed it and let it out. When you have a good cry, you release it, and the heart lightens. Heart can only open when there is so much room and grief take a lot of room in your heart so it is important to shed it out.

2. **Self-Love:** Love begins at home. When our heart is filled with love then it will radiate outwards.

3. **What goes around, comes around:** Start focussing on what you can give before what you can get. Think of what happens when you go to a party and scan who's there. Do you look there is this person I could give him my business card and maybe I could get some work out of them? Or there's that person, I need to impress them, and see how you can impress them. Or do you look and find someone sitting alone in the side, maybe they need somebody to talk to.

4. **Caring:** If we care for our children they thrive, if we care for our garden it blooms, if we care for our car, it lasts, if we care for ourselves, we are better vessels.

5. **Replace the attitude of judgement and criticism with compassion:** Notice what are the traits in the person that you are criticising, you were not allowed to do? We all have stories behind, we all have emotional ups and downs. You or me doesn't know their story, so we should not be judging them or criticising them. Maybe if you hear their story, you might feel compassionate for that person. Judgement is what we do, when we don't have understanding. Know that everybody you meet has a story.

6. **Delegate:** Devise a proper system and work flow and start

delegating the work. Make your team accountable to the task and track their growth and tasks through the systems. There are many systems through which you can track the work progress of your team.

7. **Team Building Activity:** Do certain team building activity, where you can become comfortable with your team.

8. **Gratitude Journal:** Maintain a gratitude journal, and give gratitude to all the people around you in work place for their small or big contributions.

9. **Practise forgiveness:** When we hold on to hurt, we are emotionally and cognitively hobbled, and our relationships suffer. Forgiveness is strong medicine for this. When life hits us hard, there is nothing as effective as forgiveness for healing deep wounds.

10. **Rewards and Recognition:** Start appreciating people at your workplace. You can also have some awards defined for the highest performer of the month or rising star, or special appreciation award etc. We all like to be appreciated and being recognised for the good work.

11. **Benefits of your Product/Service:** List down all the benefits of your product or services and see how these benefits can

solve your clients' problems and pain. Don't try to sell your product or services, but educate them and speak to them with the conviction that you have the power to help them.

12. **Network:** Connect with more and more people and take an initiative to introduce yourself first. The networking skill can be learned through practice.

13. **Colour:** Green colour makes you feel empathetic and peaceful.

14. **Seed Mantra:** Chant the seed mantra "YAM"

15. **Gemstone:** The stones for the heart chakra are emerald, jade and tourmaline. They help to clear blockages in the heart and to grow love and compassion.

16. **Affirmations:**

- I am worthy of love.
- I love easily.
- I hold myself and others in compassion.
- There is an infinite supply of love.
- Love is my natural state of being.
- I live in balance with others

Chapter 12

VISHUDDHA CHAKRA
THROAT CHAKRA

Chakra 5	
Vishuddha Chakra	English Name: Throat Chakra
Vishuddha Meaning	Purification
Location	Throat
Element	Sound, ether
Energy State	Vibration
Purpose	Communication
Devil	Lies
Development	7 – 12 years
Gland	Thyroid, parathyroid Gland
Other Body Parts	Throat, ears, mouth, shoulders, neck
Malfunction	Sore throats, neck and shoulder pain, thyroid troubles.
Colour	Bright Blue
Foods	Fruits
Rights	To speak and be heard

Understanding our Throat Chakra

Welcome to the wonderful world of sound and communication in the throat chakra. Sound is a wave, it's a vibration and everything in nature is vibrating. Every cell in your body, every heartbeat, every breath you take, every word you speak is vibrating.

Purpose

The Throat Chakra is connected to the way you express your life with utmost authenticity. It is about communicating your thoughts, feelings, and intentions clearly and accurately. The throat chakra, also known as the Vishuddha, is the place where we work on expanding our voice and the power of will. Vishuddha means purification. Our truth which can purify the situation.

Throat chakra is a place from where our creativity of inside comes out.

You are creating your reality at each moment by what you are speaking from your throat for example if I say go away or bring me a glass of water, that is the reality for that moment.

Chakra Development

The developmental stage of this chakra is when you start going to school and start communicating with other people effectively around 7 to 10 years. We learn to read books, watch films, we have discussions with friends and family, we listen to teachers, we receive instructions about the world, that expands our understanding.

All learning takes place through the realm of communication, whether it is communication with selves or communication with another.

So, if your inside was shamed or you had fear or guilt or even grief and you are not letting it out, then probably you are not letting things out in general. You have probably placed a sensory guard at the throat to check everything that comes out of you. That slows down the whole process and inhibits your creativity.

Blockages

- **Lies or mixed messages** – It's as simple as tell that person that mummy is not home, or put a smile on your face even if you are feeling sad. These are the ways we learn to lie with ourselves, then how can we be honest with other people.

- **Secrets** – Many families have family secrets or things they simply don't talk about. We don't talk about this uncle and his drinking, we don't talk about what happened to you sister, and we don't talk about our financial situation. That teaches the child not to share what's inside, and sometimes these are things that have a major impact.

If I ring a bell, it is vibrating until the strength of that striking is cancelled out. And that's natural. You want to talk and share your feeling with someone. But what happens when you can't do that? What happens when a child has gone through some abuse and trauma and there is nobody to talk to, or they are not believed or they are made wrong for saying it. Then the child learns that they can't let out what's inside.

Body is a vibrating instrument, if you have to stop the flow to yourself all the time, that's a process in music called deadening.

When we have to do that to ourselves, we deaden ourselves. We don't release and things get caught up inside and become tension and blockages. Instead of going towards harmony and ease of this chakra we go towards dis-ease.

- **Neglect** – Parents don't have sufficient time to listen to what the child has to say or express. Children also learn the process of expression when they are told by their parents constantly don't do this and that. They don't bring inside out; they don't say what they are feeling.

- **Ridiculed:** If we were ridiculed when we speak, then we don't trust that what we have to say is important. We may think nobody wants to hear what I have to say so just be quiet and sit on the side.

Chakra Blockages

People with blocked throat chakra are

- Scared to open their mouth. They feel they will look stupid
- Nobody will understand what they have to say

- Or their view or voice doesn't matter

- I won't be able to say it the way I want

- So, and so doesn't want to hear it.

Chakra Health and Balance

Excessive

- Talks too much. They dominate the conversation

- Loud

- Frequently Interrupts others

Deficient

- Shy and quiet

- Tiny and quiet voice

- Shrink and hide from the situations

Balance

- Clear and concise communication

- Good listening skill

- Clear creative expression

Exercise

Reflect and write down:

- Where in your life you are not speaking the truth?

- What are you afraid of speaking? How you have learned this fear?

- What is your need? (To be respected, listened to, not judged)

Chapter 13

THROAT CHAKRA AND YOUR BUSINESS

Is your blocked Throat chakra sabotaging your Business?

Whether it is customers you're dealing with, or clients, it is important to co create strong communication between every party in an operation. A healthy throat chakra enables smooth communication. One way to ensure strong communication in business is to manage your projects with accuracy and ease. When you manage your projects, make sure you stay organized, clear headed, and cultivate clear communication.

When communication goes awry, like the throat chakra, this incites criticism, gossip, not speaking up for an idea, or overpowering others. Watch for these signs in business, and insist on a project managing solution to get everybody on the same page.

Throat Chakra of Business consists of:

• Communications

• PR (public relations)

• Copywriting

• Client Engagement

- Employee Engagement

- Brand voice

- Integrity of word

- Advertising

- Project management

How a blocked Throat chakra affects your business -

- **Unclear about business advertisement post:** When the internal communication is weak the outer communication that you do is affected. While putting forward an advertisement a strong and clear message is required, which catches the attention of the audience. In case of blocked throat chakra, the message will not be clear.

- **Messages and emails are vague and doesn't put forward a clear message:** Concrete message is like a factsheet put to words. Whether you are communicating with your team, vendors or clients, it is vital to avoid any misunderstanding created due to unclear messages or emails. There is also possibility of your message being misinterpreted, which can bring huge consequences to your business.

- **Afraid to take customer feedback:** This is a nightmare for many businesses owner having issue with throat chakra. Going to customer for a review or feedback is all about communicating with your client. We fear they'll tell us our product or service stinks, that we're horrible people and we should never have set foot on earth.

- **You feel that your website, blogs, social media posts doesn't represent you and your business:** This happens because we are not communicating properly about ourselves and business clearly and properly to the outside world. In this digital era, our digital presence and reputation is very crucial, and if this channel of communication is not handled properly the important link of connecting to your audience is distorted.

- **Underlying tension in your Business:** Business is about involving your team to a common goal. When you play as a single player and your employees are unclear about their task and the bigger purpose of the company as a whole, then it will not lead to desired result. You are paying salaries, but not able to utilise their time and effort properly.

- **Don't initiate conversation:** In business meetings or handling difficult situations, deficient throat chakra person will hesitate to open the discussion forum.

- **Feel like your message isn't being heard:** You live in an interior world of conversation and feels that I have already communicated all that is necessary. But in fact, the person sitting at the other side of the table is still unclear what to do.

- **Lost connection with your truth and authenticity:** Vishuddha means purification. Our truth which can purify the situation. A blocked chakra means that you are disconnected with honesty and authenticity. Resulting in Lying or presenting distorted information.

How to Balance your Blocked Throat Chakra

1. **Release your voice:** "The fears we don't face becomes our limits". So, make sure you are practising the talking skill. Start with - Talk to nature, sing like nobody is listening, meditate and commune with the divine. Release your voice by practising singing, chanting.

2. **Learn to say NO:** Say "No" if something does not resonate with you. Do not be afraid to vocalize what you want, what you believe in, or who you are. We begin to face our truth and see beyond (illusion), when we vocalize our authentic self and no longer lie to ourselves. We remain clear and direct in speaking our personal truth when we say "I am not happy" or "This is who I am!"

3. **Speak with authenticity and honesty:** When we activate the Throat Chakra, we drop the façade of social conditioning and we awaken to our true human potential. Are you ready to speak out for what you truly believe? Our truth is necessary, speaking our truth changes the world. There is big cost to remaining silent. People will believe anything because we are not speaking our truth. Let people know how you feel. We can create new possibilities by uttering them out into the world.

4. Meditate: Meditation and quite time with yourself helps you to listen to your own inner voice.

5. Improve your listening skill: We have 2 ears and 1 mouth because listening is more important than speaking. Imagine the world that truly listens. Don't assume or deduce conclusions without listening to full story. Listen to listen, not to respond or react.

6. Process and Documentation: Have process flow and documentation in place. The FAQ's section of all the process needs to be in place. This will avoid any vagueness and miscommunications. Record your FAQ videos for reference.

7. Use Systems and tools effectively: There are many tools for handling the company's processes effectively. These tools assist an individual or team in organizing and managing their tasks successfully. Google sheets, google forms, basecamp, CRM tool etc.

8. 7 Cs of effective communication: Follow the 7Cs of effective communication, which are: clarity, correctness, conciseness, courtesy, concreteness, consideration and completeness. The 7 Cs of communication help leaders convey important messages that are understood easily, improving engagement and productivity.

9. **Learn the art of storytelling:** Practice the art of storytelling. There are many courses available that teaches you this skill. People forgets information and data but they remember stories. This skill will help you in your advertisement and creating an impact through your messages.

10. **Power of Journaling:** Start journal writing to record your life experiences and events. Have a conversation with yourself on a regular basis through this journal.

11. **Communication skill:** Involve yourself in communication skills workshops. Proper communication is a skill, which can be learned through practise. Just the way we learn to ride bicycle during our early days, similarly by constant efforts it is possible to improve and enhance communication skill.

12. **Participate:** Participate in discussions/forums/blog discussion.

13. **Social Media engagements:** Go to social media (Facebook, youtube, Instagram, LinkedIn) and do live videos. If you have your company's page connect with your audience by explaining them about your product/services. Connect with me to know more about this aspect.

14. **Read aloud a book:** Reading a book aloud also helps in exercising your vocal cords.

15. Mirror Activity: Prepare your introduction speech and then practise saying it loud Infront of mirror every day.

16. Seed Mantra: Chant the seed mantra "HAM" every day for throat chakra.

17. Colour: Bright blue colour creates calmness and opens you up to higher inspiration.

18. Gemstones: Aquamarine, Turquoise, chalcedony stimulates creative self-expression, intuitive understanding and absorbs positive energy.

19. Affirmations:

- I can speak my truth.
- My voice is necessary.
- My truth matters.
- I listen deeply to others.
- Creativity flows through me.
- I live in harmony.

Chapter 14

AJNA CHAKRA
THIRD EYE CHAKRA

Chakra 6	
Ajna Chakra	English Name: Third Eye Chakra
Ajna Meaning	Command Centre
Location	Between the Brow
Element	Light
Energy State	Luminescence
Purpose	Intuition
Devil	Illusion
Development	Puberty
Gland	Pineal
Other Body Parts	Eyes, base of skull, brow
Malfunction	Vision problems, headaches, nightmares
Colour	Indigo
Foods	Light Sattvic food
Rights	To see

Understanding our Third Eye Chakra

Welcome to the 3rd eye chakra, our brow chakra. Also known as, the inner eye, or "Ajna" in Sanskrit – it correlates to our mental abilities, psychological skills, intuition, having a vision, opening your imagination and how we evaluate beliefs and attitudes.

Chakra 1 and 2 are personal

Chakra 3, 4,5 are interpersonal

Chakra 6 and 7 are transpersonal

This chakra is about seeing the bigger picture. But first we have to clear our illusion and learn to see clearly.

We see with our 2 physical eyes that's like 2 petals on this chakra, but with the 3rd eye we can see what is underneath the surface of things.

Sitting between our eyes and being physically connected to the brain, this is the mind chakra. It resonates with the energy of our spirit, as well as our conscious and unconscious psychological tendencies.

This is the chakra of intuition, wisdom and our sixth sense. In our Indian philosophy, it is known as our 'third eye', which interacts with the rational mind in order to deepen our intuitive insight to see beyond the veil of illusion that is called "Maya."

Opening the mind and discriminating between thoughts motivated by strength, fear, and illusion are all challenges of the Sixth Chakra.

Purpose of this Chakra:

The Third Eye Chakra is Truth

Deciphering what we believe to be true and what is genuinely true is at the core of this chakra. Sometimes a negative memory can manifest as truth to an individual later in life. For example, if a person is made to believe he is ugly his entire life, then this can manifest as fact within his thought patterns and as a result, he will develop body dysmorphia and low self-esteem.

The Third Eye Chakra is the Foundation of Wisdom

The symbolism of the Third Eye Chakra is acquiring wisdom beyond our self-inflicted perceptions. It is breaking down stereotypes, seeing beyond the illusion of the media, and achieving detachment from societal realities.

The power of the Third Eye Chakra is witnessing your freedom beyond the realms of 'realistic illusion.'

Ultimately nothing is holding you back – it is only your mind that has power over you and if you can control the mind, you can then ascend any limitations you currently have.

Chakra Development

In childhood development this may come early, but often once the child has learned everything from the beliefs and patterns inflicted to them, they start seeing the world and the reality from the goggle's society has given it to them. They develop their paradigm and the way to live their lives through society and their education.

One of the challenges in this chakra is for the child or the budding adult is to learn to look at the bigger picture. How to live our lives to our greatest potential and find the real truth of our existence, to see the light in ourselves and see the light in each other?

The Sixth Chakra helps us to realize that not one person or social group can determine your life's path. When change is apparent, it is because of a larger karmic dynamic or chain of events that has led you up to this point and is moving you towards the next stage of your life.

For example, it may look like an individual has manipulated you into believing that you should stay in a job you dislike, but their thoughts are just an illusion about how you should live and will hold you captive for an entire lifetime.

Chakra Blockages

- **Traumatic Visual Memories** – Violent environment or emotional circumstances. Sometimes you start shutting the powers of your physical eyes, when you resist seeing something you don't like. When I see children wearing glasses, I often like to say so what was going on in your family that you don't like to see. Because of Traumatic Visual Memories we might: Repressed our memory or Disassociate from the memory. We say oh its nothing there, and it doesn't affect me.

- **Invalidation** - When your thoughts and feelings are rejected, ignored or judged, then we shut this chakra and start to invalidate ourselves. What is the consequence of that? Instead of looking at the larger vision we get into vicious self-scrutiny and self-consciousness. So, we are always conscious of how do I look, how am I moving? Instead of just being ourselves.

- **Doesn't trust Intuition:** Also, you might lose trust in your intuition and listen more to the outer world. You ignore that little voice inside and what's that trying to tell you.

Our thoughts and attitudes play an enormous role in creating or destroying the health of our bodies. Depression, for example, directly diminishes our immune system and affects our very cells from healing because the body communicates with the mind.

Chakra Health and Balance

Excessive

- **Open to any input** – This is happening and that is happening. They are kind of overloaded in psyche input
- Unable to sort out truth from fantasy

Deficient

- Blind and insensitive: Don't notice anything. They are the person over for dinner and everybody looking at their watch yawing and this person is talking on and on not oblivious to what's around them.
- Rigid Perspective: can see only one side of the story
- Denial: Can't see what's going on.

Balanced

• Good clear intuition

• Insight, you have perceptive, you see things in people

• You are able to visualize and think symbolically

• You have a good imagination

• You are able to see the vision of your life.

How to Balance this Chakra

The challenge of this chakra is illusion. Illusion about how something should be, instead of seeing how it is. We might be fixated on our body being 10 kgs thinner or attached to what I call perfect pictures. One thing about perfect picture is that they are never in real time – (I should have this kind of relationship, or this kind of job or this kind of body and it keeps you from seeing what you do have).

Another aspect is always seeing what's wrong and failing to see the light and beauty in yourself and others. And when we overcome this illusion, we have

• Clear perception

• Awakening

• Insight

Chapter 15

THIRD EYE CHAKRA AND YOUR BUSINESS

Is your blocked Third eye chakra sabotaging your Business?

The third eye represents intuition, imagination, and direction. The third eye of business is your business development. Where do you want to go? Where do you want to grow? Do you want to expand your horizons, expand your business and assimilate into another market? What are your businesses fullest potential, and how are you going to get there? When you have an unbalanced third eye, you can suffer from lack of focus, and the inability to visualize your future. Leaders with high Ajna activation follow their inner voice and act with higher levels of integrity.

The Ajna Chakra of your Business consists of:

- Long-term vision

- Business growth

- Focus

- Balance between intuition and strategy

- Imagination

- Business ideas

- Openness to new, unknown possibilities

How it affects your business

- **Have trouble making decisions:** For making any decision, you need focus, clarity and an ability to visualize the future perspective of things. Blocked 3rd eye chakra will give you a foggy picture and because of this you will fear making decisions.

- **Visions aren't coming true:** A dream is a vision of how you desire the future to be. After coming up with a clear vision, you need to take steps every day to make it a reality. But what if your visions are hazy? When we are not able to visualize clearly, whatever results we get will definitely be not be in accordance to our dream, because we ourselves are not clear what do we exactly want.

- **Lack of clarity and imagination:** Through awakening your third eye chakra you gain a great ability to intricately perceive life and its infinite potentials. This experience of expanded and integrated consciousness gives rise to innovative interesting ideas and thoughts which can manifest in various forms. If you feel like you have trouble with visualization, creative problem solving, artistic creation, and maybe even get bored easily this can be because you have an underactive imagination. I find it quite exciting to know that no one lacks the ability of a wonderfully vivid imagination, we are innately creative beings, sometimes it is just a matter of identifying and unblocking, awakening, and releasing the natural energy that wants to flow uniquely within and through each of us.

- **Feel foggy in your business goals:** Not able to visualize the long-term goals for yourself and your business is a sure sign of a blocked 3rd eye chakra and mental confusion. Not sure what you want in 5 years, 10 years? The picture is very vague in your head. Unclear about your business long term strategies.

- **Difficult to connect with your intuition:** Instinct is also known as the sixth sense which is the innate wisdom, we have that affects our response to various life experiences. Feeling disconnected from intuition and instincts can have you feeling very confused about your life purpose.

- **You experience unexplained depression, anxiety, and feelings of sadness:** The pineal gland plays a role in the production of the hormone called serotonin. Serotonin is also known as the happy hormone which affects our brain chemistry and has a direct impact on our moods and emotions. A pineal gland or third eye which is not functioning in a balanced manner can impact your moods intensely. A blocked third eye can, therefore, be a cause of some of your unexplained anxieties or feelings of depression.

How to Balance Third Eye Chakra

1. **Visualization Guided meditation:** There are many guided meditations available online which can help you to increase your visualization power. Regular practice will surely benefit you.

2. **Colour and art therapy workshops:** Working with color is a powerful lifestyle practice that you can use every day to create magic in every aspect of your life. Color can be used to bring your heartfelt dreams alive, to energize, to heal, to relieve stress, and to give you a clearer direction for moving forward towards your self-development goals.

3. **Create a vision for your life:** What do you really want? The world is changing at a high speed. The power is coming to common people, to impact the world and change the lives. And then use your throat chakra to tell the vision. Inspire the society, uplift them. When a building is made before that a blueprint needs to be there to structure the material into existence. Without the blueprint it would be difficult to create the building. Similarly create a blueprint of your life. Where you are and where you want to go. The problem is we are sleep walking through the life, taking challenges as and when it comes. We don't have any fixed agenda of our lives.

4. **Seek Professional Guidance:** There is a systematic process to make long term goals and plans. Seek a help of professional to make long term goals. Break down your goals into small doable pieces and take action on 1 task a time. If your business feels stagnant and you haven't grown in a while, it might be time to look for more options like hiring a business development consultant.

5. Time Management skill: Time management principles also will help you to be more productive and gives you a sense of achievement. Plan your day and task properly to avoid mental confusions.

6. Take proper Rest: Proper sleep and food is crucial for getting in touch with your intuition and judgement

7. Choose to see the positive: Pay attention to negative dialogue with others and yourself. Remember brain needs a 5:1 ratio of positive to negative things to retain a sense of positive well-being. Its human tendency to remember even 1 criticism and forgets about 99 appreciations.

8. See the bigger picture: One illusion that we are living into is that we are separate from others. I am separate from you. Illusion of separation. As we see the big picture, we see that we are really all one.

9. Use the Power of Journaling: Reflect on what you see or don't see. Make use of your visualization to seeing things beyond. Instead of seeing roadblocks see it as stepping stone to success. Possibility to what you can create. I M Possible. Journaling your thoughts on a regular basis will give you lots of insights. You will be able to catch your thoughts.

10. **Practise coming to stillness:** Our general world is a reflection of our thoughts and patterns. In order to see that reflection carefully, you will have to become still and notice it. Example you go to a camping and early in the morning you sit watching the lake, you can clearly see the reflection of the mountains or the sky in the lake. But when the ducks wake up or boats start humming or children start playing in the lake the reflection of the same mountains becomes dim and there are waves in there. Similarly, all during the day there are stuff in your life that needs your awareness and they scream at the top of their voice – look at me, look at me. So, in meditation or stillness we are quieting the mind and the reflection we see is not distraught. We can see things clearly.

11. **Take a perspective outside yourself:** Get into their shoes and understand others. The more we increase our perspective, the more we increase our understanding of the world.

12. **Seed Mantra:** Chant the seed mantra "AUM".

13. **Colour:** Indigo colour provides your mind with inner calmness, clarity and depth. It strengthens, heals and opens up to subtle levels of perception.

14. **Gemstones:** Lapis Lazuli, Indigo blue sapphire stimulates intuition, clarity of perception.

15.Affirmations:

- I see with clarity.

- I pay attention to my intuition.

- I have a vision.

- I focus my attention to see clearly.

- I value my insights.

- I am open to the wisdom within

Chapter 16

SAHASRARA CHAKRA
CROWN CHAKRA

Chakra 7	
Sahasrara Chakra	English Name: Crown Chakra
Sahasrara Meaning	Thousand-Fold
Location	Top of head
Element	Thoughts
Energy State	Consciousness
Purpose	Understanding
Devil	Attachment
Development	Throughout life
Gland	Pituitary
Other Body Parts	CNS, Cerebral cortex
Malfunction	Depression, alienation, confusion, boredom, inability to learn
Colour	Violet, white
Foods	Fasting
Rights	To know

Understanding our Crown Chakra

Our lower chakras are the stepping stone to our higher consciousness. The root that is deep allows the plant to grow tall. Then those roots need to be watered and water needs to move all the way through. We need to harness the sunlight. That's your power to bring that fire into the belly and into your core. And we want to blossom out from the heart. After that we attune in the throat; we see our way in the sixth chakar. **But here is a question who is it that's doing all of that, who is it that lives inside us, seeing things, hearing words, living in our body, running the show of our life, making our decisions. Who is that and how do we know? The answer is – Our Consciousness, that is doing all that.** Consciousness that sees, hear and turns those words into meaning. Consciousness that loves and feels the connection with everything else. Consciousness that knows how to take action. consciousness that feels and operates our body. The seventh chakra relates to mind, especially the awareness that makes use of the mind.

All acts of creation begin with the conception. We must first conceive an idea before we enact it. This begins in the mind and then descends through other chakras into actual manifestation.

So why is it important to come to consciousness?

Our mind assimilates experience into meaning and constructs our belief systems. Matrix structures are created from the meaning we derive from the experience. They become our personal belief systems and the ordering principles of our lives. If we repeatedly fail, and we tell ourselves that it means we are stupid, we eventually generate a belief in our own stupidity. These belief systems form a matrix into which all other information is funnelled.

The relationship between meaning and belief system is so strong that if some piece of data doesn't fit our inner matrix, we might say," I don't believe you, and discard the information entirely.

Different people derive different meanings from the same experience, because they carry a different belief system.

This is one of the traps of the mind. How do we take in new information and expand our horizon, if we reject anything that doesn't fit our current inner belief system?

Chakra Development

This one is not so much about the developmental stage as we are constantly learning about the world, processing our thoughts, studying, taking information and making our own internal roadmap of the world around us. But there comes a time when we grudge away from our childhood, when we grow and go out on our own. And at that time, we begin to make our own world. It might not be that same one that your parent thought. You might have a change in the point of view.

We question and we start to create our own world view. Our bigger picture, understanding of how everything goes together. There is enormous expansion of consciousness through learning, and then we go out and explore the world.

Sometimes during the process, we develop higher

consciousness, that is we receive wisdom or experience that is beyond ourselves.

Some people find it difficult to understand the higher power, which is understandable. Your first experience of higher power is your parents. When you were little infant, and you didn't know much about the world, they were your guidance, supporter, they were the one who watched out for you. And if you couldn't trust them for some reason, maybe they were not in the right frame of mind, or they didn't give you the guidance that you needed, or maybe you didn't really trust their wisdom, then you must have closed that crown chakra to being able to download and trust that higher power.

Chakra Blockages.

Excessive

- Live up in your head and gather too much information
- Disconnected with yourself
- Difficult in focussing

Deficient

- Too anchored in the mundane world
- Sceptical about the spiritual world
- Learning difficulties
- Close – mindedness and rigid belief systems.

Balance

- Connected with something larger than yourself
- Intelligent – able to think clearly
- In your wisdom – awareness

Chakra Health and Balance

So, as we go from roots to up, we go from one single body to multitude of thoughts.

We go from finite to infinite. The main challenge of this chakra is attachments. While attachment is necessary to make commitments or keeping focus in the lower chakras, example attachment to your job, that's normal. But there are other kinds of attachments that restrict the flow of liberating current. Maybe you are too attached to what people are thinking about you, maybe you are attached to understanding why and figuring things out. Maybe you are attached to looking good, youth, money and things. Whenever you are releasing your attachment, you are freeing your attention from that attachment.

When we talk about 7th chakra we also talk about Kundalini, which is prana, energy force or shakti. We have knots in our chakras that is called granthis and that keeps the energy from passing through. It is a powerful force and rises chakras by chakras up the spine and rises up to the crown. It's a process to be done under guidance. We will not cover Kundalini here. Currently as an Entrepreneurs we have to see how to balance our chakra and align it for our growth and success.

If you struggling with a question like what to do in your life, or something about your relationship, health just put out a question to the universe. Be open to receiving the answer. Look out for answer. I do that all the time, a particular page from a book would open up, an advertisement would come, a friend would just call up to discuss the same problem, or I might get a dream related to the same. Just be open to receive the answer. Don't expect an answer right away.

Chapter 17

CROWN CHAKRA AND YOUR BUSINESS

Is your Blocked Crown Chakra sabotaging your Business Growth?

The crown chakra is the energy centre located just above your head that is responsible for connecting you, as an earthly human being, in physical form, to source energy—God, the universe, the divine, spirit, consciousness, however you choose to define and refer to it, it's that higher power that is the loving source of all that is.

When this chakra open, and you're openly communicating with that source energy, you have this beautiful feeling that everything is always going to work out for you. You don't question what, you accept it and keep moving forward without worry, fear or anxiety because you have an undeniable faith that you're love and are being taken care of.

I love moving through my days knowing that everything is always working out for me. It's a peaceful feeling. But the one thing that has blown my mind since taking steps to open my crown chakra, is the **"information downloads"** that happen.

Information downloads are when you are sitting quietly with your thoughts (meditating or just being present) and suddenly you get a genius idea (or surge of ideas) that just come from out of the blue. You know the thoughts aren't yours, but they're really good so you take off into action mode to do something with them. These thoughts are the answers you've been seeking to a problem or question, or perhaps the information to connect you to a life-changing opportunity. This book, was the result of "downloaded information" that came to me after a meditation session.

In nutshell Crown Chakra of Business consists of:

- Giving back to the people, society and environment

- Co-creation: Not feeling better than others but a complete balance of infinite abundance

- Collaborating with other companies for a cause

- Spiritual side of your business: A healthy crown chakra implies a presence of complete peace and wisdom

- The larger purpose of your company

- Faith and trust in your vision

Signs of Blocked Crown Chakra

- **Scepticism:** Not trusting that everything will work out for you. When things are going well also, you may have a fear that the bottom is going to drop at any minute and that the goodness won't last.

- **Worried about what others think:** Do you find yourself constantly worrying about what others think of you? Are you worried that people might be judging you and what you are doing? If this chakra is blocked then it's easy to get caught up in feeling worried about how you may look, or what others think of you.

- **Over-thinking:** You are anxious about tomorrow and spend a great deal of time fearing (or thinking) about all the negative outcomes that are possible. The to-do list gets longer and longer, without any concrete action.

- **Resistance:** Feeling like no matter how hard you "try" you have to keep pushing harder. Nothing in life seems to come easily.

- **Feel disconnected from your Business:** Business is a reflection of you. When you are disconnected with self, it's difficult to put your heart & soul into the business.

- **Your inspiration is blocked:** You find it difficult to trust the higher powers, which is our source of inspiration. Many of your ideas goes unnoticed or it gets filtered through your funnel system of belief, which says "It is not possible", or "I will not be able to do or achieve it".

How to Heal your Crown Chakra?

1. **Meditate:** Try doing meditation to develop the practice of slowing down and being with your thoughts. Just be your silent witness.

2. **Spiritual Retreat:** Take time out to go on any spiritual retreat, where you are disconnected to the world. Your phone is switched off, and you are there with yourself only. I plan spiritual retreat for entrepreneurs, so that they connect with self for the future growth. Mail to me to know more (coach. manika@gmail.com)

3. **Maintain Journal:** Journal your day-to-day events and see it from a third person perspective.

4. **Read:** Read more books to open your perspective of the world.

5. **Carry a diary:** Carry a small diary every time with you. Whenever an idea pops up, open it and immediately note that idea. Ideas coming to you is a signal that these needs to be given attention to. At the end of the week, you can sit by and analyse all the ideas gathered one by one.

6. **Gratitude:** Once you inculcate the attitude of Gratitude, you will start noticing and experiencing miracles in your life. Treat yourself as scared, treat ground, food, people as scared divine beings. We are here together on this planet to create miracle. We change ourselves from inside by remembering that we are a god or a goddess walking on this earth to bring blessings.

7. **Attachments:** We are attached to lots of things in life, which doesn't allow us to see the bigger picture. Below is the list of

few attachments that I have listed. Mark the one, which you think you are attached to. Ask yourself: What can I do to release these attachments?

People	Staying young
• Places	• What other people think
• Possessions	• Knowing the answers
• Your home	• Suffering
• Money	• Freedom
• Looking good (physically)	• Spiritual practice
• Pleasure, Self- gratification	• Success
• Power	• The past
• Being right	• The future

8. Colour: Violet colour dissolves blockages and brings about a transformation of mind and soul.

9. Gemstone: Wearing gemstones like Amethyst, diamond dissolves fear, disharmony, congestion and blockages in life and provides you with new energy and protection for contemplation, meditation and inspiration.

10. Affirmations:

- I am awake and aware.
- The world is my teacher.
- I am guided by higher intelligence.
- I am guided by inner wisdom.
- Divinity resides within.
- All is one

HOW ALL THE CHAKRAS FLOW IN SYNCHRONY

Thank You for sticking through the learning and continuing to hunt for the treasure. Let's learn how to bring heaven down to earth and live the life of your dream. So, in the journey upward, we did a lot of healing on ourself. We cleared our chakras and took steps to reach to our higher awareness.

Now it's time to make it practical, to apply it in your life to create the life you want, the life of your dreams.

Why is this Smooth Flow Important?

In moving up - We go from fixed earth current to moving and flowing water current, to radiating fire to air which is light and invisible, to sound, to light to consciousness.

In downward current – we are taking the higher consciousness to create a vision for life to talking about it, to bringing it to our relationships, we are doing something about it, we are moving things around, and finally, we are manifesting our dream.

Both current are always working together in our chakra system. We are taking energy in from our thoughts, and we are bringing it down. We are always evolving and moving out of limitations and expanding.

The two currents pass each other and create a vortex, spinning and revolving and creating a wheel of energy called Chakras.

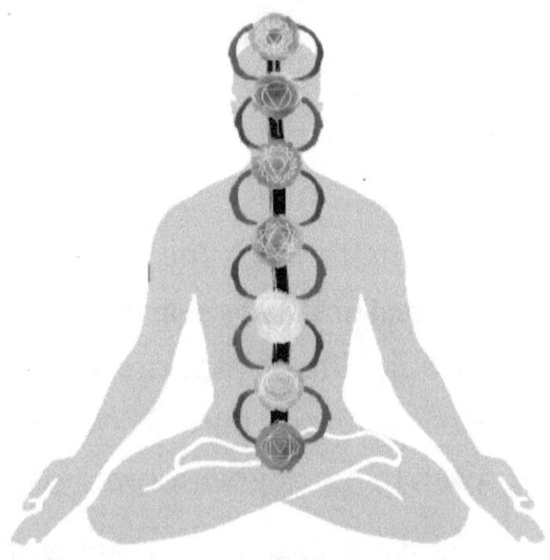

In lower current, you have things that you can feel, see and touch. In higher chakra, you have more of a liberating current, where things are a little vague.

How do downward Manifesting current works?

When you go in downwards current, you feel resistance. Because when you go from a plane of less density to a plane of more density, you experience a little resistance.

When we are at the thought plane and create some imagination, and that imagination needs to be told to somebody, we need to be more specific. We have to clearly define what we are thinking. So, everything needs to be a little clearer and more concrete. It's natural to feel a little more resistance. And because of that resistance, we experience more blockages in our system.

So, let's apply these principles to something like building a house.

When you build a house, first you have to have an idea to build a house. You have to set an intention that I want to build a house.

Then you have to think about where do I want to build this house, for how many people, how many bedrooms, would it be a simple house or a luxurious house.

All creations start with a thought. Its starts with an idea. We get lots of ideas every day.

But when you begin to take the downward current, things start to take shape. You say I am going to set an intention. Now I am going to begin building a house.

Setting an Intention and having an idea is the 7th chakra.

Consciousness Creates - Everything that comes into creation starts with an idea.

The next step is you start to visualize your house. What kind of house do you want it to look like? What do you want the house to look like when you walk into the doors? Maybe you start visiting other people's houses to see how they build their homes. Understand their architect. Collect ideas through magazines, pictures, internet. This takes place through visual frames.

That is the 6th Chakra, Chakra that sees.

Vision Vitalizes

Now you got a clear idea of what you want; you will go and talk about it, probably with an architect. How many square feet, budget, material, bedroom will I have?

Communication Catalyses

When you talk about your idea, you may find that the other person has a solution or can refine your vision, gives feedback, and get clearer and more specific by talking about it.

Love Launches

We want to treat all our relations with love and positive regard. Any dream that you want to create, you need to build lots of relations—relationships with architects, banks, real estate agents, contractors and workers, neighbours.

3rd part. This is the hard part as it's now action taking time.

Power produces

You have to empower yourself to get things done. That's how you are going to produce the results that you need. Prioritize your plan if you look at the whole project once it can be overwhelming. But if we break it down into manageable chunks and empower ourselves to overcome our obstacles, we can get things done.

Fun part 2nd Chakra – Pleasure Pleases

To do all these things, you got to make it fun and enjoyable for yourself and the people involved in the project. People are attracted to what is beautiful, what is enlightened. That will keep you on track.

When you put your whole heart, soul, your passion and enthusiasm into the work,

you start to get results. You start to see the first shoots of that plant coming out. At that point, we get all the more excited and passionate; we say, wow, it's working. You get the first review on your book; you get your first client who tells you that they have a wonderful experience. Things come down to gravity and come together.

After all the hard work, we finally came down to manifesting plane root chakra. Matter Matters.

It's important that you cut the board in the exact same size, or you cut the nails in a very specific size.

Calculations and specificity come into the picture. You also put things on the calendar and say that Wednesday at 10:00 a.m. I will make these calls. We have to be specific in making an appointment with the ground to really ground things into space and time.

And if you do that, you get to have your dream in its finished form.

If all our Chakras are balanced and working in synchrony, the idea will be manifested for us. If one of the chakras is blocked or unbalanced, the idea will get stuck and will not materialise. I have seen many times that people have many ideas popping up in their minds, but they never come true. Somewhere or the other, it gets stuck.

Balance your energy and balance your life. We all are sent on this earth with an advantage of human life, where we have the power to create things and create our own life. Knowing about the Chakra system is the first step to knowing and understanding your power.

Own your Power!!!!

Chapter 19

WHAT DO WE DO?

Most of the time, people ask me, **"Is it true or real?** Now, this has two answers: Yes and No. I have explained all the logical reasoning behind the concept. **Yes,** it is true for you, if you believe it. And **No**, it is not true if you believe that ways - *The glass is half empty or half full, depending on how you look at it.*

We spend all our lives being a victim of our situation. We blame ourselves, luck, other people, government, competitors or circumstances for all our troubles.

We keep creating the same type of results by thinking the same kind of thoughts. But there is no rule book that says that we can't change our thoughts, patterns or our belief system.

If as a child we were taught that the world is a frightening place, then everything we hear and do will fit into this belief system. The same is true for don't go out at nights, don't trust strangers as many people are cheaters.

And if we were taught that the world is safe, then we would hold this belief. There will be no problem in accepting that love is everywhere, people are friendly, and I always have whatever I need.

Almost all of our negative and positive programming was accepted by us by the time we were seven years old. Our life experiences are generally based on the belief system we have accepted about ourselves. The way we treat ourselves now is usually the way we were treated when we were small. The person you are scolding every time for any mistake is a small child who is living inside you.

Whenever you get angry at yourself for being fearful and afraid, think of yourself as being that little child. If you had a little 3-year-old child in front of you who is scared, what would you do? Would you scold him, or would you reach out your arms and comfort him so that he feels safe? When you were a child, maybe the adults around you didn't comfort you. But now you are an adult in your life, and if you are not comforting the child within you, that is indeed very sad.

Whatever happened in the past is over. Now you have the opportunity to treat yourself the way you wish to be treated. A frightened child needs comforting, not scolding. Scolding yourself only makes you more scared. The child within feels the same way now, the way we felt when we were belittled when we were young. Be kind to yourself. Begin to love and approve of yourself. That's what that little child needs to express itself at its highest potential.

Through this book, I have tried to explain how our core programming was developed and what you need to do to balance yourself now.

But knowing is not enough; you have to apply and practice the techniques regularly.

How to Change

"We are what we think all day long". You can train your mind to be a Master or your Servant. You have the power to train or untrain your mind to become what you want it to be. The way your mind is operating now is only a habit, and with conscious practise any habit, can be changed.

The thoughts you choose to think create your experiences in life. If you believe that it is hard to change a habit or a thought, then of course, it is difficult for you. But if you believe that I am in command of my thoughts and will change the way I think, then it will be easier for you to follow through.

Suppose you allow your child to stay up as late as he wishes, and then one day you make a decision that from now the child has to sleep at 9:00 every night, what do you think the first night will be like?

The child will rebel against this new rule and may kick and scream and do his best to stay out of bed. If you surrender to his tantrums at this time, the child wins and will try to control you forever.

However, if you calmly stick to your decisions and firmly insist that this is the new bedtime. The rebellion will lessen. In probably few nights, the new routine will be established.

It is the same thing with your mind. Of course, it will rebel at first. It does not want to be re-educated. But if you stay focussed and firm, the new way of thinking will be established in a very short time. And you will feel so good to realize that you are not a helpless victim of your thoughts but rather a master of your mind.

It is my wish that these topics "Chakra Management", "The power of thoughts" etc should be taught in schools. Our education system should also focus on important subjects like - How the mind works, how to handle finances, how to invest money for financial security, how to create and maintain self–esteem and self-worth.

Just imagine what a whole generation of adults would be like if they had been taught these subjects in school along with their regular curriculum? We would have happy people who feel good about themselves. We would have people who are comfortable financially and enrich the economy by investing their money wisely. They would have good relationships with everyone and would be comfortable with the role of parenthood and then go on to create another generation of children who feel good about themselves.

Thank you for staying with me till the end of this book. Wish you Health, Wealth and Prosperity.

Exercise

Here we are again. Look at the self-assessment and become aware of which chakras has improved or needs more attention.

POST-ASSESSMENT

POST-Assessment: Overall Chakra Health

Now you have understood the chakras and its disbalance, it's important to gauge your chakra health. The post-assessment below is helpful for two reasons:

1. It will help clarify what areas you need to focus on.

2. It will help you understand which areas you've developed.

There is an assessment at the front of the book as well, rate yourself again here to see how much you have grown. Then, calculate the difference of your pre and post assessments.

If there are areas where you still feel stuck, areas that didn't change that much, then you know where you need to do deeper work, or apply the practices longer or more diligently. Don't beat yourself up about it, just keep up the efforts. They will pay off in the long run.

Instructions

Use the rating scale below to rate yourself on each statement.

Not at all	A little	Sometimes	Often	Most of the Time
1	2	3	4	5

First Chakra: Root

1. _______ I have trouble finding or holding my ground.

2. _______ I'm not at ease in my body.

3. _______ I have health challenges.

4. _______ I hate to exercise.

5. _______ I struggle with food, diet, or weight.

6. _______ I never seem to have enough money to live comfortably.

7. _______ I feel disconnected with nature and the earth.

First Chakra Total = _________

Second Chakra: Sacral

1. _______ I have trouble knowing what I feel.

2. _______ Some people think I'm overly emotional.

3. _______ I find sexuality to be challenging for me.

4. _______ Life just isn't a whole lot of fun.

5. _______ My body doesn't move very freely.

6. _______ I have trouble knowing what I want and need.

7. _______ If I do know what I want, I'm scared to ask for it.

Second Chakra Total = _________

Third Chakra: Solar Plexus

1. _______ I get overwhelmed by life's challenges.

2. _______ I have trouble bringing tasks to completion.

3. _______ I'm not sure what my purpose is.

4. _______ I feel intimidated by others.

5. _______ I struggle with low energy.

6. _______ I'm not very good at setting boundaries.

7. _______ My will gets distracted and goes in many directions.

Third Chakra Total = ________

Fourth Chakra: Heart

1. _______ I have trouble finding or maintaining intimate relationships.

2. _______ I am critical and judgmental of myself.

3. _______ I am critical and judgmental of others.

4. _______ I feel isolated and alone.

5. _______ I am shy about reaching out.

6. _______ Other people take too much energy from me.

7. _______ I hold a lot of grief in my heart.

Fourth Chakra Total = ________

Fifth Chakra: Throat

1. _______ I have trouble speaking what really matters to me.

2. _______ I tend to interrupt others when I should be listening.

3. _______ I have trouble getting my ideas across effectively.

4. _______ I wish I could be more creative.

5. _______ I often feel out of sync with others.

6. _______ I find it difficult to express myself in writing.

7. _______ Sometimes I don't know what's true in what people tell me.

Fifth Chakra Total = __________

Sixth Chakra: Third Eye

1. _______ I have trouble trusting my intuition.

2. _______ I have trouble imagining things different than they are.

3. _______ Sometimes I ignore that little voice inside.

4. _______ I rarely remember my dreams.

5. _______ I don't have a guiding vision for my life.

6. _______ I have trouble visualizing what I want.

7. _______ I don't really notice details around me.

Sixth Chakra Total = __________

Seventh Chakra: Crown

1. _______ I try to meditate but don't stick with it.

2. _______ I don't feel very connected to any kind of spirituality.

3. _______ I find it difficult to learn new things.

4. _______ I often think I'm just not smart enough.

5. _______ I am wary of new ideas.

6. _______ I'm not sure of my purpose.

7. _______ I don't know what I'm here for.

Seventh Chakra Total = _________

Scoring

All Chakras Total Score = _________

"Most of the time" in all columns (worst score) would be 5 x 49 = 245

"Never" in all columns (best score) would be 1 x 49 = 49

If you scored anything between about 100 and 245, it means there's room for improvement.

Connect with Author

Direct access links to Author

Website: www.manikasingh.com

(For various video courses offered by Manika Singh, please visit the mentioned website).

Facebook Page: https://www.facebook.com/successhabitscoach

Instagram: https://www.instagram.com/manika.ksingh/

Email Id: coach.manika@gmail.com